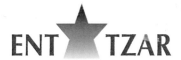

Otolaryngology ST3 Interview Guide
for National Selection

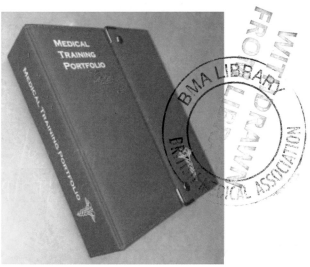

Ricardo Persaud, Amir Farboud, Konstantinos *
Tahwinder Upile

Foreword by **Professor Henry Pau**
MD FRCS (ORL-HNS)

1st Edition 2013

First published 2013 by FASTPRINT PUBLISHING
Peterborough, England.

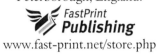

www.fast-print.net/store.php

OTOLARYNGOLOGY ST3 INTERVIEW
GUIDE FOR NATIONAL SELECTION
Copyright © Ricardo Persaud, Amir Farboud, Konstantinos
Argiris & Tahwinder Upile 2013

A catalogue record for this book is available from the British Library

ISBN 978-178035-550-4

An environmentally friendly book printed and bound in England by
www.printondemand-worldwide.com

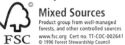

This book is made entirely of chain-of-custody materials

OTOLARYNGOLOGY ST3 GUIDE FOR NATIONAL SELECTION

(with questions and answers)

CONTENTS

Preface

For all those wanting to specialise in Otolaryngology, performing well at interview the first time round has never been more important. Not only are the number of National Training Numbers in Otolaryngology reducing each year, but the introduction of a negative grading system based on length of training means if candidates do not perform well on their first attempt the chance of securing a position the second time round becomes much more challenging. Consequently it is imperative that all trainees who attend the national selection day for ENT prepare extensively.

The impetus for this book came from the constructive feedback received from ST3 delegates who attended our mock interview courses. Our aim is to provide a unique insight into the national selection process and in doing so allow the readers to understand what will be expected of them on the big day. This book is also intended to provide a framework for which prospective candidates can base their revision around and is therefore an obvious starting point for those contemplating the selection process. It should be stressed that the tips, knowledge, questions and answers provided within this book will help the candidate to prepare, but in order to do exceptionally well further reading is required and above all plenty of practice to refine your interview technique and oral-aural presentation.

Finally, remember the more work and effort you put in now the more successful you are likely to be. We wish you all the very best and look forward to meeting you at our ST3 mock interview course (for further details visit www.enttzar.co.uk)

Ricardo Persaud, Amir Farboud, Konstantinos Argiris and Tahwinder Upile - **January 2013**

Extended Prologue

And words of encouragement

If you are reading this, you are probably a Core trainee (CT2 or CT3), a Locum Appointment Trainee (LAT, LAS), an old style SHO, or even a doctor from oversees hoping to become a higher surgical trainee in ENT. What you are about to do is probably the hardest task you will ever face. To be honest, if I had taken the selection process more seriously at the beginning, read more books, went on a few more courses, then it wouldn't have taken me so many attempts to get my National Training Number (NTN). Hindsight is a powerful thing, and we hope in this book the experiences and mistakes of those who have achieved their goals can be shared, and the process can be simplified and demystified. I remember walking around with a folder of loose paper full of guidelines, useful tips on management and clinical governance, but it never felt complete. I would go on a course and add to my big folder, but it was still lacking something. This guide serves to bridge that gap and give a generous coverage of all the main topics that could be encountered in National Selection, in a concise format. The book has been broken up into one introductory chapter and 6 other chapters which are intimately related to the 6 interview stations that you will encounter at the English National Selection. Although the other National Selection programs are not covered specifically, you will find an abundance of useful and indeed applicable information for those programs within these pages.

How do I know this you may ask? Well, through my own endeavour, and attempts at applying, I have an intimate knowledge of the processes involved, what the interviewers expect and what to say and what not to say and do. This book was conceived as a way of consolidating that knowledge, and by asking the best and the brightest what they thought and incorporating their views. By doing this I believe that we have produced the most comprehensive guide to this application process currently available. This book may also be useful junior Foundation trainees, CT1, Registrars and Trainers, who would like to gain an insight into the national selection process in England.

If you are making a committed application to an ENT ST3 position, you are in a group of highly competitive individuals in the top 0.5% of the UK's educated elite, and so if you have any doubt in your mind about your capability and strength of character, then you would be wise, and indeed sensible to re-consider, because the road is long and hard and requires tough thick skin. The process of National Selection will either make or break you. If you feel you have a weak portfolio or CV, then bow out early, make the most of your opportunities to strengthen your application, re-group, and apply again the following year, "What doesn't kill you makes you stronger" as the old saying goes. Going through this process will mature you as an individual until slowly you will become the semi-finished article, someone ready to take on the role of the SPR, and progress to becoming a Consultant.

Above all else, when applying for National Selection, take the opportunity, to learn and reflect on your past performances, and to then move forward and improve yourself. Approach your interview preparation like you would an exam, put pressure on yourself to achieve goals in terms of learning and knowledge. The difference here is, exams you can take again, here you have one shot, so make it a good one!

I would like to acknowledge my family, especially my wife Charlotte and mum for endless tea and snack production that kept me fed and watered through the exam and interview preparation, and the endless hours of viva practice from my wife who is now an expert on the National Selection process. Without family and friends my achievements would not be possible.

Mr Amir Farboud
2nd year ENT SpR
Wales Deanery

Foreword

It gives me great pleasure to write the foreword for *Otolaryngology ST3 Interview Guide for National Selection*. Over the recent years I have noted the increased competition for ENT training places and the improved preparation and calibre of potential candidates. After reading this manuscript I am confident that its contents will significantly improve the chances of anyone attempting to obtain an ENT training number at National Selection. The main authors include two ENT Consultants and Specialist Registrars who have successfully navigated the ST3 national selection pathway. This book has solid information not only for potential ST3 candidates in general but also for anyone preparing for ENT postgraduate examinations and vivas. It highlights succinctly the behaviours, skills and knowledge necessary to succeed at ENT National Selection and to practice as a Registrar. I have no hesitation in recommending that you read this well-organised guide early, in order to start moving towards a fruitful ENT career.

Professor Henry Pau *MD, FRCS (ad eundem), FRCSEd (ORL-HNS)*
Visiting Professor, University of Loughborough
Consultant ENT Surgeon, University Hospitals of Leicester
Honorary Senior Lecturer, Leicester University Medical School
Research Lead, ENT SPR Training Program, East Midlands Deanery
Medical Council Member, Patient Liaison Group, Royal College of Surgeons of England
ENT Educational Lead, Undergraduate Medical Studies, Leicester University Medical School.

Contributors

Konstantinos Argiris

Specialist Registrar
KSS Deanery
Chapters 1 - 6

Suki Ahluwalia

Specialist Registrar and President of AOT
London Deanery
Chapter 4

Ashwin Algudkar

LAT London Deanery
Chapter 1

Samuel Cartwright

Specialist Registrar
KSS Deanery
Chapter 7

Amir Farboud

Specialist Registrar
Wales Deanery
Chapters 1, 3 and 7

Bhavna Gami

Academic FY2 Surgery
NW Thames Foundation School
Chapter 7

Hiten Joshi

Research Fellow
East Anglia Deanery
Chapter 5

Nicholas Hamilton
Specialist Registrar
London Deanery
Chapters 4, 6 and 7

Sonna Ifeacho
Specialist Registrar
London Deanery
Chapter 3

Robert Nash
Specialist Registrar
London Deanery
Chapter 7

Ajiya Olakunle
Specialist Registrar
East Anglia Deanery
Chapter 4

Ricardo Persaud
Locum Consultant ENT Surgeon, Head and Neck
Surgeon, University Hospitals Leicester (LRI)
Chapters 1-7

Peter Radford
Specialist Registrar
Oxford Deanery
Chapter 3

Sunil Sharma
Specialist Registrar
London Deanery
Chapter 6

Anna Slovick

Specialist Registrar
London Deanery
Chapters 1, 2 and 7

Costas Stamataglou

CT3
London Deanery
Chapter 7

Tahwinder Upile

Hon Senior Lecturer, University of London
Chapters 1-6

'The greatest glory in living lies not in never falling, but in raising every time you fall.'

- Nelson Mandela

Acknowledgements

Many thanks to all those who made this book a reality, especially all the contributors and Hannah Applin. We are also very grateful to Professor Narula for his unstinting support and encouragement and to all the ST3 delegates, ENT Consultants and SpRs for permission to include their photographs in this book.

Dedications

To all ENTTZAR Ambassadors:

Past, Present and Future

Chapter 1

Introduction

In this introductory chapter, we provide an overview of surgical training in Otolaryngology in the United Kingdom, examinations to be taken, national selection for higher surgical training, the marking scheme and a personal account of a candidate who successfully navigated the ST3 national selection pathway.

1.1 UK surgical training in Otolaryngology

Surgical training in the United Kingdom has changed significantly over the last 5 years and this has impacted both core and higher surgical training. Further changes may take place in the next few years. At present the standard career pathway for ENT consists of 2 foundation years training (FY1 and FY2), 2 years core surgical training (CT1 and CT2) and then 6 years of higher specialty training (StR) in ENT, leading to the award of a Certificate of Completion of Training (CCT). After registering with the General Medical Council, CCT holders may take up a Consultancy position (Figure 1).

Figure 1 The pathway from medical student to Consultant

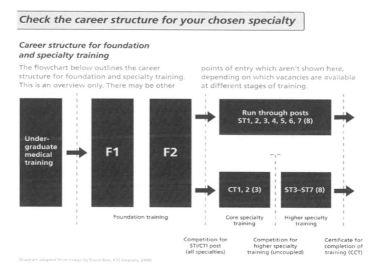

Upon completion of the primary medical degree (e.g. MB BS), two years of foundation training (FY1 and FY2) in a mixture of medical and surgical specialties (usually in the form of six four-month rotations) would need to be completed. After foundation training, you then be required to undergo a two year core surgical training program. This is a competitive application process as the quality of the trainees is quite high, in that the majority of them are extremely focused and aware of the commitments that are necessary for career progression. Moreover there has been a decrease in core surgical training numbers recently, further augmenting the competitive nature of the process. Once accepted, however, the allocation of specialty rotations within core surgical training is usually based on performance at the national selection interview. In the London Deanery, three four-month rotations are designated for the CT1 year according to the trainee's interview performance at the core training interview (trainees will rank the offered list of rotations beforehand). For the CT2 year two six-month rotations (occasionally in the same specialty at the same hospital) are allocated on the basis of a "matching" interview/OSCE which takes place during the CT1 year. Some deaneries alternatively offer a set two year rotation for trainees, and invariably try to theme their rotations before hand. It is therefore advisable for candidates to familiarise themselves with the process of post allocations before applying by checking each Deanery website.

The London Deanery also offers a CT3 or "post core training fellowship" year for trainees who wish to gain more experience at SHO level in a given specialty before applying (or re-applying) for higher training. There has been some debate about whether a three year core training programme for all trainees would be a better platform for higher training than the current two years. This would permit a generic first year, allowing ample time for trainees to access appropriate training for their chosen specialty in the second and third years. There has been support for this suggestion but it has also been met with resistance elsewhere as it would lengthen the course of training by a year. At present in England only two years of core surgical training (with sufficient experience in the specialty of choice) are mandatory before progressing on to higher surgical training.

Once core surgical training has been completed, a candidate can apply through National Selection for a numbered training post. To be eligible for higher training in ENT, the necessary examinations [MRCS + DOHNS, or MRCS (ENT), or MRCS + MRCS (ENT)] in conjunction with a minimum of six months experience in ENT must have been completed. Each of the United Kingdom countries currently runs their own National Selection process with National Selection in England now in its fifth year.

Higher training consists of a six year programme during which Specialty Registrars must cover the curriculum. The progress of trainees is recorded on the Intercollegiate Surgical Curriculum Project (ISCP) website and annual checks on progress [Annual Review of Competence Progression (ARCP)] must be satisfactory. A similar process also occurs through core surgical training, so trainees should be familiar with the whole process when entering higher training. Upon successful completion of higher training, including passing the intercollegiate FRCS examination, candidates are able to apply for a CCT. Before authorising the award of the CCT, the Joint Committee on Surgical Training carries out a number of checks (including a check on the minimum numbers of index operations that a trainee is expected to have carried out as lead surgeon). CCT holders are then eligible to apply for consultant posts; however, a fellowship is often undertaken prior to the commencement of a consultant job.

At present a significant number of posts CCT ENT surgeons are unable to find a UK consultant post because the expansion of UK ENT consultant jobs did not occur. This is being addressed by reducing National Training Numbers. In England only 32 and 34 new numbered trainees were appointed through National Selection in 2011 and 2012, respectively. It is thought that it will take six years before the reduction in the numbers of new higher specialty trainees has a significant effect on the number of surgeons gaining CCT.

1.2 ENT examinations for core trainees [DOHNS, MRCS, MRCS (ENT)]

There are currently three examination options available to trainees hoping to pursue a career in ENT: The Diploma of Otolaryngology - Head and Neck Surgery (DOHNS), the

Membership of the Royal College of Surgeons (MRCS), and the Membership of the Royal College of Surgeons in ENT [MRCS (ENT)]. To progress to higher training in ENT trainees must be in possession of the MRCS and DOHNS diplomas or the MRCS (ENT) diploma.

DOHNS

The DOHNS examination has been available since 2003. It replaced the Diploma in Laryngologist and Otology that had been available since 1923. The examination is made up of two parts. Part 1 is a two-hour written paper consisting of multiple true/false questions and extended matching questions (Em's). There are approximately 140 questions in total. Once Part 1 has been passed, a candidate becomes eligible to take Part 2. This takes the form of an Objective Structured Clinical Examination (OSCE) with up to 28 stations of seven minutes each, taking just over three hours in total (with rest stations). Usually six of the stations are manned and involve performing an examination on a patient, taking a history, explaining a disease, consenting for an operation or performing a basic procedure (e.g. - flexible nasendoscopy). The remainder of the stations are un-manned and involve interpreting and answering questions related to photographs, scans, audiograms, instruments or anatomical specimens. During Part 2 of the examination, answers will have to be written on an answer sheet and then placed in a folder provided to every station. At the end of the examination the folder will be collected.

The DOHNS became "intercollegiate" in 2008 (London, Edinburgh and Glasgow) and, since 2012, also includes Dublin. Part 1 of the examination is held simultaneously at all centres three times a year with Part 2 also being held three times a year but rotating through the four colleges. College regulations recommend at least six months experience in ENT before attempting Part 1 of the examination. At present there is no limit on the number of attempts a candidate may require to pass the constituent parts of the DOHNS examination.

MRCS

The intercollegiate MRCS has been available in its current form since 2008. As with the DOHNS, it consists of two parts. Part A is made up of two two-hour written papers (one morning and one afternoon). The first paper is titled "Applied Basic Sciences" and consists of 135 single best answers questions (SBAs). The second paper (more clinically orientated) is titled "Principles of Surgery-in-General" and consists of 135 EMQs. Once Part A has been passed, the Part B of the examination can be taken. Part B is an OSCE with 18 stations of nine minutes each, taking just over three hours in total (with rest stations). Unlike the DOHNS every station has at least one examiner present. Twelve of the 18 stations are taken by all candidates with the remaining six stations allocated in accordance with what the candidate has chosen from four specialty context areas (three from the following are chosen with decreasing preference: *head and neck*, *trunk and thorax*, *limbs including spine* and *neuroscience*). College regulations advise that part B of the examination should not be attempted during foundation year training and at present only four attempts at part B are permitted.

MRCS (ENT)

The MRCS (ENT) diploma has only been available since 1st August 2011. To be awarded this diploma the candidate must have passed both the MRCS Part A and the DOHNS Part 2. After obtaining a pass in the MRCS Part A, current regulations state that a total of four attempts at any combination of the MRCS part B and the DOHNS Part 2 are permitted in order to be awarded the MRCS or the MRCS (ENT). If a candidate who has passed the MRCS Part A goes on to pass the MRCS part B and the DOHNS Part 2, he/she will be awarded both the MRCS and MRCS (ENT) diplomas. Details of the examinations can be found on the Intercollegiate Examinations website. Contact details for the examination department of each of the Colleges are given below.

1.3 National selection for higher surgical training

Application for higher surgical training in ENT in England occurs once a year, and a similar selection process occurs in Wales and Northern Ireland. In Scotland, however, a run-through system operates where core surgical training and higher training are combined, notably, trainees from the rest of the UK are still able to apply for ST3 posts in Scotland.

The English applications are computer-based and run by the Yorkshire and Humber Deanery. Both the application process and the application form itself are similar to that for core training; therefore a trainee is not faced with any particular unknowns at this stage. In 2011 application, most of the information required consists of a review of the trainee's curriculum vitae (CV) with particular reference given to the achievements gained during core surgical training.

To be eligible for appointment to higher training, trainees must have a minimum of six months' experience in ENT (12-18 months being ideal) and have successfully completed the MRCS and DOHNS examinations or the MRCS (ENT) examination. Further credit is awarded to trainees who have had experience working in the specialties allied to ENT such as: plastic surgery, oral and maxillofacial surgery (OMFS), A&E, GP, neurosurgery, upper GI surgery, ophthalmology, cardiothoracic surgery, ITU, paediatrics, paediatric surgery and audiological medicine (not lower GI or orthopaedics).

In 2011 there were 140 applicants for 32 National Training Number Posts in England. There was a similar number of applicants in 2012, 34 National training appointments were made, including two new numbers in Yorkshire and one Defence Medical Service number. On both occasions, around 15 Locum Appointments for Training (LATs) were made after awarding national training numbers.

National selection assessment takes place over three days (usually in April) with the first day used to train the selectors and other two days for actual interviews. The candidates usually go through six different stations, viz:

1. **Portfolio**
2. **Clinical Scenario**
3. **Communication**
4. **Clinical Skills**
5. **Managerial**
6. **Structured Interview**

In this guide, we address each station separately as a chapter. Our main aim is to elucidate the essential core material necessary to optimise your chance of scoring maximum marks in the interview. Past questions and answers are also provided.

1.4 An overview of the marking scheme for ST3 national selection

The marking scheme for ST3 National Selection is constantly evolving. However, in 2011 and 2012, marks were allocated for global assessment of your Portfolio, structured answers, fluency and logical thinking in all six stations. The Portfolio station usually carries more marks than any other station as points are allocated for both the Portfolio *per se* and the Portfolio interview. In 2012, a disproportional amount of negative marks (20) were allocated for having too much ENT experience (>30 months), presumably in an attempt to get rid of 'the lost tribe'. At the end of each chapter, we have included a brief synopsis of the marking scheme relevant to the station, based on 2012 National Selection Process.

Top tips:

The assessors will be across the desk from you and will have very strict criteria of what they expect you to cover in your answer. If you deviate from the topic, they cannot give you the marks that you deserve. Try and use buzzwords like "governance" and "teamwork" carefully. Try to be as analytical as possible, making it look as though you have thought about your answer, rather than just rambling on. At all times try to personalise your answer with specific examples.

1.5 Personal experience of the ST3 national selection process

My background

Becoming an ENT surgeon was my goal since medical school. Ever since completing two ENT Special Study Modules in my penultimate and final years, and feeling inspired by those academic around me, I just knew that ENT was right for me. Following my graduation, I consciously endeavoured to experience rotations that contained ENT within my Foundation School in order to strengthen my ENT skills and also to use it as a medium through which I could make an informed choice about my future career path. Upon completion of my Foundation training, it was clear in my mind that the only specialty I wished to pursue was ENT. I consequently opted for an ENT themed rotation during my Core Surgical Training attaining the maximum experience I could (i.e. 18 months) as a Core Trainee. In the next few sections I will describe my experience from the process of National selection.

Getting off the mark as a CT2

It would be fair for me to say that by the beginning of my CT2 year I was not competitive enough to get an ST3 post. From early on, however, I organised my preparation by splitting it into essential exams, CV-related achievements, demonstration of ISCP progression, portfolio preparation and interview preparation. Moreover I tried to become fully aware of the ST3 process timeframe as set out by the relevant deanery website. Undoubtedly tackling all these elements successfully would require much hard work and excellent time management, but by staying positive and enthusiastic, I maintained motivation and remained focused on the target that was the ST3 number. Familiarising myself from the start with the person specification was of great value; however, my first aim was to complete my examinations, so that I could later devote my focus and attention on the application. I also took an honest look at my CV and highlighted areas that needed to be addressed urgently. My personal areas of focus were quite a few, those being publications, presentations, teaching and audits; so I demonstrated initiative by carrying my own projects and organising my own teaching course for medical students. Fortunately my efforts resulted in a few publications (including publication of audit as first author), presentations and a full cycle audit. Throughout the year I also tried to keep up to date and expand my knowledge by reading journals and attending relevant courses. I also focused on my ISCP progression by trying to create a reasonably strong logbook and finishing my Work Based Assessments (WBA's) in advance to avoid last minute stress, in particular nearer the ARCP time. By addressing all of these targets, I believe I was as well prepared as I could be for the first stage of the ST3 recruitment process - the on-line application.

On-line application

Before the actual application was open, I ensured my details and all the other relevant information had been registered on-line (Intrepid ^{TM}). This means that when the ENT application became active its completion was not as time consuming as it would have potentially been. The first few pages of the application enquired about previous ENT jobs and relevant experience as well as whether the appropriate qualifications (i.e. DOHNS and MRCS for ENT) were attained. For me, the application was very straightforward to complete, especially as I had made efficient use of the preceding time ticking all the relevant boxes. By the closing date of the application I felt confident with what I had submitted and immediately began preparing for the interview and organising my Portfolio (before I heard from the deanery) so I would not lose any valuable time.

Portfolio and interview preparation

There was roughly a 50 day timeframe from the closing date of the on-line application to the actual interview dates. Within this time, and by having saved a few extra days of study and annual leave. Moreover I had also taken the liberty to book myself on two interview courses (a generic one and an ENT specific one) both of which were closer to the interview date, and proved ultimately to be invaluable. The details of my portfolio preparation can be seen in the relevant Portfolio Chapter (please see Chapter 2). In summary, I took it extremely seriously, paying particular attention to its appearance and layout. Fortunately, I had most of the validation documents required which saved me a lot of time. With respect to the interview preparation I tried to split it into six distinct categories; classic interview questions, clinical governance and management questions (including difficult scenarios), audit and research (including teaching), clinical questions (including a lot of ENT theory revision), clinical skills (i.e. examinations and procedures) and communication skills. During this preparation I thankfully received an interview invite but not knowing the status of my application did not in any way, change my preparation. If anything, it motivated me further for the big day!

The Big Day – The Interview

Being geographically a fair distance away from the interview venue, I decided to stay there the night before as I did not wish risking any commuting mishaps on the actual day. It was a pleasure to meet a few friends on arrival that were in the same boat as I was and it also gave me the opportunity to relax a bit and think about something other than interviews. After an understandably restless night, I woke early the next day. I began to mentally prepare myself and headed down to the interview area, bringing with me all the documents that had been requested by the Deanery. For some reason however they did not have time to check mine and asked me to come back down after the interview. I was not extremely happy about that but tried to remain calm as we approached the interview rooms. There was a deadly silence between us candidates as we came across some of the examiners that were preparing themselves for the next set of interviews while having a cup of coffee. It was time though to focus and psych myself up for the big moment. We all handed in our portfolios and then were placed outside a door which had an A4 sized piece of paper, indicating the type of station and a preparatory statement. There were a total of six stations all of which lasted ten minutes. By the time the first bell rang and I entered the room, time lost its meaning. It was just about tackling each question or situation as well as I could. The hour quickly passed and I welcomed the well-earned feeling of relief one it was all over. As there was no room for predictions, I collected my portfolio and went to complete the administrative component of the interview. As soon as that was done I was then homeward-bound with a glimmer of hope, awaiting the results that would by revealed around ten days on.

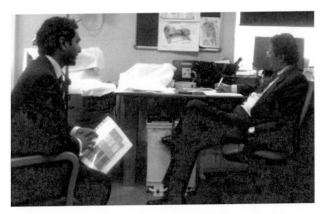

Figure 1.1 Professor Narula grilling a ST3 candidate on ENTTZAR ST3 interview course 2011 (do not be surprised to see Professor Narula at National Selection 2013 - therefore dress up, sit up, speak up and then shout up, and finally no brown shoes please!)

Result

I had planned to go on holiday during the week the results were supposed to be published. Feeling extremely uneasy, I would check my on-line application every hour until I suddenly noted an offer. In a flurry state of anticipation, I read the offer for an ENT number and could just not believe my eyes. It was undoubtedly one of the biggest days of my life when I saw that all my hard work had paid off. I had been successful.

References

The Royal College of Surgeons of England Examinations and Assessment Department

> Webpage: www.rcseng.ac.uk/exams
> Telephone: 020 7869 6281
> Email: exams@rcseng.ac.uk

The Royal College of Surgeons of Edinburgh Examinations

> Webpage: https://ubis.rcsed.ac.uk/examinations.aspx
> Telephone: 0131 527 1600
> Email: examinations@rcsed.ac.uk

The Royal College of Physicians and Surgeons of Glasgow Surgical Examinations

> Webpage: www.rcpsg.ac.uk/Examinations/Surgical/
>   Pages/ex_surgical_homepage.aspx
> Telephone: 0141 221 6072
> Email: exam.office@rcpsg.ac.uk

The Royal College of Surgeons in Ireland Postgraduate
Examinations

> Webpage: www.rcsi.ie/index.jsp?p=100&n=240
> Telephone: +353 1 402 2100
> Email: exams@rcsi.ie

- ❖ Selection. TL Lesser. ENT & Audiology News September/October 2011 Vol 20 No 4 p. 50-52
- ❖ http://www.mmc.nhs.uk/pdf/PS%202011%20ST3%20Otolaryngology_1.pdf
- ❖ http://www.yorksandhumberdeanery.nhs.uk/specialty_recruitment_2011/specialties/ENTST3NationalYHDLead.aspx
- ❖ Royal College of Surgeons of Great Britain and Ireland: welcome to the MRCS and DOHNS (www.intercollegiatemrcs.org.uk)
- ❖ The MRCS (ENT) Exam. G John. ENT & Audiology News September/October 2011 Vol 20 No 4 p.62-64

- • Training in ENT. J Davis. ENT & Audiology News September/October 2011 Vol 20 No 4 p.57-58
- • www.entuk.org/career_advice/ accessed via the world wide web on…

Chapter 2

Portfolio Station

2.1 Overview

At the beginning of the National Selection process, you will be asked to hand in your portfolio. For about 20 minutes, an assessor will scrutinise it against a set marking scheme without you being present. The assessor will probe into the accuracy of the evidence provided and your probity, in addition to evidence of your achievements stated on your application form. This process is followed by a portfolio interview, where you will be asked questions related to information inside or outside your portfolio. It is important that you have evidence for everything you put down on your application. This is of particular importance, especially when trying to back up your answers in front of the interviewers in the Portfolio station. Finally, the portfolio station is one of the few stations that has personalised questions, as opposed to generic ones, and this enables you to demonstrate your unique achievements, qualities and enthusiasm for ENT. In this chapter we provide details on how to prepare the ideal portfolio as well as details on the actual portfolio interview. Past questions and model answers are also provided.

2.2 The Portfolio *per se*

With the recent changes in surgical and medical training within the UK, a new component has been introduced to aid the process; the creation and maintenance of a portfolio. The portfolio can be seen as a self-made professional document containing every aspect of your career ranging from university degrees and evidence of progression within the training pathway, down to teaching experience and other extracurricular activities. Simply put, the portfolio can be seen as your professional life. The importance of this document cannot be overemphasized, as it is one of the means by which you are assessed in order to progress through every stage within the extremely competitive training pathway. Besides giving you the opportunity to demonstrate all of your related achievements and experience, further desirable aspects can be shown. Without a doubt it is an organisational skill exercise and the successful trainee should be able to amalgamate every aspect of his/her training in a clear and concise manner. Moreover, as surgery is about precision and attention to detail there is no reason why this should not be applied to your portfolio. Finally, the creation of a good portfolio requires other skills, namely IT skills, giving it that extra edge.

Top tip

Success is about taking the portfolio extremely seriously as it is a vital document which takes lots of time to reach top class standard.

Becoming a strong candidate

It is imperative that you focus on all aspects of your development before even thinking about preparing a portfolio. Consequently, you should strive at becoming as competitive as possible, therefore maximising your scores at the first stage of national selection. A very useful document that you should familiarise yourself with early in the process is the person specification. This document sets the scene of what is expected from you and should be used as a guide. A serious candidate though should not only be looking at the essential criteria but also the desirable ones. In combination with this, regardless of how strong you are at the beginning of the CT2 year, it would be advisable to pay particular attention to preparing an up-to-date CV at that very point. It is very important to be strict with yourself, paying specific attention to the weak areas; most commonly being publications, national presentations, prizes and full cycle audits. Initially, most trainees feel daunted by the amount of work that needs to be done; but with a lot of hard work, an attitude to make the most of each rotation, some intuition and a bit of senior help, anyone can progress considerably. As a rule of thumb (from personal experience), you should spend every day of your CT2 year until you have completed the online application form on some activity that will strengthen your CV. Reassuringly, most candidates become more productive once they become core surgical trainees. In fact, many gain most of their achievements in their final year. Once you have maximised your chances from an academic (publications, courses, research, teaching, audit) and surgical perspective (ISCP and logbook), have updated your CV and sent your application, the focus needs to be shifted onto building your portfolio while preparing for the interview as well. It should be stressed here that you should give at least 4-6 weeks preparation time for the portfolio. In the remainder of this chapter the steps to building the perfect portfolio will be outlined.

Top tip

Success is about constantly striving for improvement and good timing

First impressions do count

Even in our everyday encounters, first impressions undoubtedly play a major role in how we unconsciously approach somebody or something. It is for this very reason that you should pay specific attention to the external appearance of your portfolio (Figure 2.1). There are no specific rules on how this can be accomplished; however, the aim should be to make it stand out in a positive way inviting itself to be opened. Bear in mind the examiners and the number of portfolios they go through during national selection, and then consider the importance of an eye catching one. A good starting point would be paying attention to the quality of the binder itself. There are many available options on the market and these can be easily purchased online. Many of these can be customised to your specific needs therefore you can experiment with colours and pictures quite easily. Suffice to say that with some creativity, beautiful portfolios can be made. In addition, some information can be added on the portfolio itself. Even though there are no guidelines on this, your name and some indication that it is a portfolio are essential. Your GMC number could also be added. It is important to stress at this point that examiners would spend literally a split second scanning the portfolio from the outside. It therefore has to be professional as if it really means business, and have the appropriate information on the outside with a reasonable font size. By taking pride and demonstrating creativity a winning portfolio can be made.

Top tip

Success is about paying attention to details.

Figure 2.1 Examples of two well-presented Portfolios

Example 1

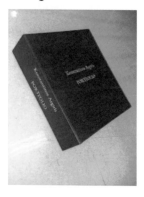

Example 2

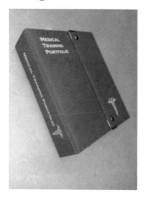

Portfolio content

Trainees are often unsure about how to section their portfolio as there is no available advice or a standardised approach on this matter. Nonetheless, in some circumstances candidates that are offered an interview are specifically requested to arrange their contents in a particular way. For example, at the ENT interviews of 2011, candidates were asked to have a section in the front of the portfolio with all the validation documents arranged in a specific way. In effect, all the statements that were made by the candidates at the application stage needed to be verified. Needless to say that in such cases you should adhere to what has been requested and *not* do something different. Clearly, a portfolio is not only comprised of these validation documents, and further sections can be added. It is important here to take a step back and think about what the portfolio actually needs and what the examiners would be interested in seeing. For example, the examiner would be more interested in seeing a certificate of a teaching course you organised as opposed to a scuba diving certificate you may have obtained during your holidays in Cuba! Below is a suggested example of portfolio contents (Figure 2.2) and can be used as a guide.

1. Degrees
2. Evidence of Training
3. Qualifications
4. Courses
5. Publications and Peer Review
6. Audits
7. Posters and Presentations
8. Prizes
9. Core Surgical Training Portfolio and Surgical logbook (summary)
10. Foundation Training Portfolio
11. Research
12. Teaching
13. Curriculum Vitae
14. Appendix (detailed logbook, teaching feedback etc)

Top tip

Success is about predicting what the examiners want to see.

Figure 2.2: Examples of good organisation of the content page

Example 1

Contents

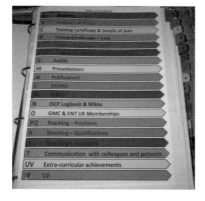

Example 2

Collecting the Portfolio information early

Putting together a portfolio is a time consuming task so it is advisable to start collecting all the appropriate paperwork early, so that valuable time can be spent in the final few weeks on the layout of the portfolio and the actual interview itself. This may sound straightforward and unnecessary, but it is remarkable how many trainees delay doing this and end up getting stressed-out, awaiting key letters/e-mails just a few weeks before their interview date. From the start of the CT2 year (or equivalent), to when the up-to-date CV has been prepared, you should ensure proof of participation/completion of all the activities you have been involved with (e.g. audits, research, presentations etc). This is often the most arduous and time-consuming part as it may entail contacting old consultants/supervisors. To avoid unnecessary chasing with any project/activity you are involved with, make sure you obtain a signed certificate or e-mail as proof as early as possible.

Top tip

Success is about proving all of your achievements and limiting any unnecessary sources of stress

Organisation of Portfolio

Once the binder and contents have been completed and all the information is collected you will have to think about the actual layout of the portfolio. Once again there are no specific rules on how this can be accomplished. You may have some ideas on achieving this as what is described here is only a suggestion. Nevertheless, it would be advisable to make the first page of the portfolio the contents page. It would be a good idea to experiment and use some IT skills here by making it appear a bit more interesting, with some colour perhaps. You should remember however that on the one hand it would be preferable to be eye catching but on the other hand should contain the basic information that is easily legible at a single glance. Following this the portfolio contents will need to be split with dividers. It is worth bearing in mind that if numbered dividers are used, the same number should be placed in the contents page. You could also use a colour theme, but this should only be seen as an addition rather than a way of splitting the contents. Moreover, you should ensure that the dividers are clearly visible and extend beyond the core document, making the examiner's life easy while scanning through the portfolio. It would be a major mistake here to assume that by simply adding all the information in the relevant sections the job is complete. Examiners are bombarded by so much information in each portfolio and it is the candidate's responsibility to make this process as simple and pain-free for them as possible! A nice way of tackling this is by adding a section specific contents list just after the section divider (Figure 2.3). By doing this, the examiner will be able to immediately go to a specific section e.g. audit, scan through all the documents and then be able to study them individually. One could also try and maintain the colour theme here, making it all that more eye catching. A very easy way of making this contents list is by copying and pasting the relevant section from your up-to-date CV. That way the information displayed will be in harmony and consistent with the CV. Tables may also help to consolidate information and make information easily accessible. (Figure 2.4).

However, in future, you may be asked to organise your portfolio in line with the marking scheme to make it more convenient for the assessor.

Figure 2.3 Examples of sub-division of content within the body of portfolio

Example 1

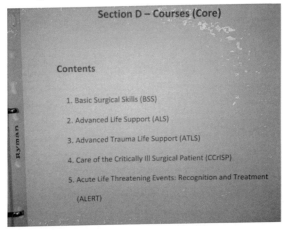

Example 2

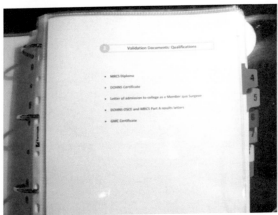

Figure 2.4 Tables may help to make information look more organised

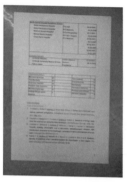

The final stage of portfolio preparation

The final stage of preparing the portfolio is probably the most pleasant one as you can see all of your work as a junior doctor comes together. Before doing this however you should purchase good quality clear plastic pockets that can be easily placed in the portfolio. The golden rule here is that the examiner should *not* have to take the contents out of the pocket. All the information should be clearly presented, like a book, unless the examiner specifically wants to go through one of your projects in some depth. When putting the portfolio together you should ensure that the sequence of information matches the section specific contents list. From that point onwards the presentation of the portfolio information depends on its type. Degrees, evidence of training, qualifications, courses, prizes, teaching certificates or any other certificates can simply be placed in sequence as no other accompanying document are required. Audits, publications, presentations and posters nonetheless should be approached differently. The front page should have a copy of the relevant activity demonstrating the title of the project and the names of the participants and on the back should be the proof (signed document, e-mail, letter of acceptance etc.). The examiners will therefore see everything they wish with two glances. All the information here however should match the information present in the section specific contents list and even more importantly, the information present in your application form! The Core Surgical Training information including all the learning agreements and work based assessments (WBAs) should all be displayed in separate pockets. All of these, as with the most recent documents of your progress and training, should be freely available to the examiner. In order to demonstrate further attention to detail, you may want to make a contents page for all the WBAs, making it easy for the examiner to scan through these. Clearly a candidate who can demonstrate some variation in the themes of these assessments will be seen more favourably as opposed to the one who has 12 CBDs on glue ear! The foundation year documents however can be placed in a more compact way as the examiners are unlikely to want to see these. With respect to the logbook, a summary of the operations should be placed after the Core Surgical Training portfolio. A detailed signed logbook however should be placed in the appendix. Teaching feedback should also be placed in the appendix as it is unlikely that the examiners will go through these during national selection (they should be available however, should they wish to see them). Finally, the CV can be put in a separate binding folder within the portfolio, just in case the examiners wish to read it.

Top tip

Success is about making the examiners' life easy by using a high quality professional printer to obtain good quality photos.

Summary of Portfolio

- Your portfolio is *your* life and therefore the most important document you can prepare
- Take your time and pride in preparing it. It is a fun process!
- Demonstrate your academic skills to their full extent but also your creativity, attention to detail and organisational skills
- When preparing your portfolio, always keep in mind who you are preparing it for (i.e. the examiners)

2.3 Portfolio interview

Having had a chance to look through your portfolio, the assessor may be keen to clarify some issues of concern. For example, you may be asked if you personally completed your audit cycle and to explain exactly what you did. Assessors are particularly keen on errors, no matter how small. There is no excuse for spelling or grammatical errors. Career progression became part of both the short listing and interview marking scheme in 2011, in an attempt to mitigate previous bias against core surgical applicants. Therefore you may be asked about your career progression, explaining any gaps in your training, clinical experience or skills. The following section highlights some of the typical questions and model answers.

2.4 Questions and answers

Question 1. *What is the point of a portfolio?*

To answer this, you need to be familiar with the Intercollegiate Surgical Curriculum Programme (ISCP), Postgraduate Medical Education Training Board and GMC Principles. In essence the portfolio is the written representation of the trainee, and is the means by which evidence is provided in terms of career progression, personal development and the attainment of appropriate competencies. You should therefore speak about all of these things, and that would take the form of completed audits, research experience, relevant courses attended, an up-to-date logbook and an adequate number and quality of work-based assessment. The portfolio however does go deeper that this as it is also a tool allowing for self appraisal – thus leading to your own learning/development. Finally, it is the means by which formal learning agreements are made between the trainer and trainee.

Question 2. *Are there any weaknesses in your portfolio?*

This is always a difficult question to answer. The examiner knows that every candidate has weak points and they are not expecting flawless individuals. Tackling this question effectively requires insight into your own weaknesses while making it sound positive at the end e.g. "I have minimal experience of research, however, I am familiar with the principles and intend on pursuing it actively during my training."

Question 3. *How does your portfolio differentiate you from others?*

Any trainee should have at least one unique selling point and should be prepared to elaborate on this. Typically such questions are answered by either describing some research that has been published, answering a pertinent question in ENT practice, a description of any other qualifications of relevance (MSc, PhD), or electives in ENT etc.

Question 4. *How have you used feedback in your training?*

The fundamental principle of the ISCP portfolio is that trainees seek feedback from their trainers and subsequently aim to improve their practice. In essence this forms the foundation of sound and safe clinical practice. However, this can be expanded to other activities such as teaching others, actively seeking formal feedback and then subsequently changing the session to address anything raised. Teaching is also good as it can be used to provide evidence of a number of qualities judicious to a trainee.

Question 5. *How can optimal training be achieved in the context of the EWTD?*

This is alluding to the fact that training is competency based. As a result, in order to achieve this you should talk about maximising learning opportunities by attending consultant led ward rounds, MDT meetings and departmental teaching/M&M days while endeavouring to gain as much operative experience as possible. Attending targeted courses allows improved understanding and application of learnt skills in the operative setting with greater confidence. Finally, you must seek perpetual assessment and feedback through CBDs, PBAs, CEXs and e-PATs, and learning from mistakes that have been made. Undertaking fellowships and observerships may also significantly optimise training.

Other past questions include:

1. 'What has been your best teaching experience?'
2. 'Talk to me about surgical/ENT training'
3. 'Why haven't you got any extracurricular activities in here?'

4. 'Did you actually present all the oral presentations that are in here?'
5. 'What do you think of work-based assessments?'
6. 'What do you think are the disadvantages of WBAs?'
7. 'What is the difference between summative and formative assessment?'
8. 'What makes you stand out as someone who wants to do ENT?'

In conclusion, good preparation is essential to performing well at interview. The groundwork, however, will have been done long before. This is never more true than for the portfolio station as it is time consuming not only putting it together in a way to visually impress the interviewers, but the substance must stand up to scrutiny. We therefore repeat urge you to 'start early', as this will negate some of the potential concerns nearer the interview.

Figure 2.5 Professor Narula lecturing on ENTTZAR Portfolio Preparation Event 2011

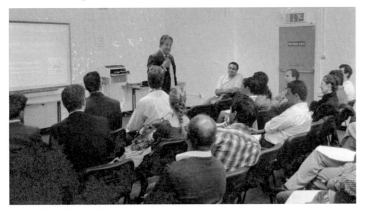

2.5 Marking scheme

In 2012, the total number of marks for the Portfolio station was 110 (Portfolio *per se,* 100 marks; Portfolio interview, 10 marks). With regards to the Portfolio itself, marks were allocated for specific events such as academic awards, extra academic qualifications, extra-curricular activities, courses attended, teaching experiences, publications, audits and presentations, log book, time spent in ENT and allied specialties (including GP, ophthalmology and A&E, but not lower GI surgery or orthopaedics) as well as general presentation of the Portfolio. In the portfolio interview section marks were set aside for familiarity with your own Portfolio, its limitation, awareness of the characteristics of a good leader and insight into one's own behaviour and practices. Approximately ten percent of the total marks were allocated for global assessment of portfolio layout and presentation plus global assessment of interview answers.

Chapter 3

Clinical Scenario Station

3.1 Overview

This station is designed to see if you are going to be a safe Specialty Registrar by testing your response to a clinical scenario. This is likely to be an emergency situation and the interviewers want to see that you make calm reasoned decisions in an ordered fashion. You must be aware of your own limitations and make it clear when you would call for help. Whilst seated outside the station you will be presented a page outlining the clinical scenario. This may include radiology images or clinical photography. The material will be present in the interview room too but make sure you read it thoroughly. Once you are sure you've read it, read it again. It's all too easy to miss obvious pathology or misinterpret the question when you are under stress. On entering the station the interviewers will introduce themselves and then ask you to talk about the case. They may start by asking you to identify the problem or ask you to dive in with your management strategy. After you have given your general answer follow up questions will test your knowledge further. In this chapter we provide some general advice on the clinical scenarios including the positive and negative indicators. We have also selected the seven most common scenarios you are likely to be asked about in this station. Model answers to the scenarios are included.

3.2 General advice on clinical scenarios

- Stay Calm! Give your answer in a good steady pace – they are selecting people who are good under pressure.

- Identify emergency situations by making a bold statement at the beginning: say "this is a potentially life threatening problem", "this is an airway emergency", "this is a vision threatening condition". The interviewers then know that you know it's a serious case.

- Don't skip ahead. Never start by saying "I would firstly perform an emergency tracheostomy" – quickly assess the patient along standard algorithms before jumping to management.

- Remember ALS, ATLS, and APLS – starting with these algorithms (where appropriate). Know the doses of medications suggested by these algorithms, know how to calculate paediatric resuscitation fluid volumes etc.

- Don't be afraid to say you'd call for help. Many cases would not be appropriate for an ST3 registrar to manage alone. Be prepared to phone your consultant for minimum advice but if you need them to come into the hospital say that's what you would ask for. The most useful bit of equipment in the A&E resuscitation room is the telephone!

- Part of your real life management involves consenting patients for emergency procedures, talking to parents/relatives and communicating with other colleagues. Remember to state that you would do these.

- Clinical Governance: this might be relevant to the case e.g. recording an adverse outcome from a procedure for morbidity and mortality purposes or filling in a clinical incident form. Stating that you would do these things completes your answer.

- Refer to your own experience. Nothing beats personalisation to let the examiners know that you have dealt with similar cases. "When managing a case similar to this I found…".

3.3 Positive and negative indicators

Assessors have strict criteria of what is safe and unsafe behaviour. How you tally up with regards to positive versus negative indicators (Table 3.1) determines the score you get for the station. The stations are all scored from 0 to 5 depending on how many negative indicators there are. Zero is unappointable with many negatives, 1 is poor, 2 is area for concern, 3 is satisfactory, 4 s good and 5 is excellent with no negative indicators. Below is an example of indicators from a neck trauma station.

Table 3.1 Positive and negative indicators relevant to clinical scenarios

Positive indicators	Negative indicators
• **Takes history from patient and witnesses** • **Structured approach to assessment (ABC and survey for other injuries)** • **Assesses airway appropriately** • **Initiates appropriate supportive measures** • **Appropriately considers cricothyroidotomy and tracheostomy** • **Involves other staff appropriately e.g. anaesthetists and senior**	• Fails to take history from patient and witnesses • Unstructured approach to assessment (ABC and survey other injuries) • Does not assess airway appropriately • Fails to instigate supportive measures • Does not involve other staff appropriately • Fails to arrange investigations appropriately

ENT staff

- **Arranges appropriate investigations**
- **Formulates appropriate management plan**
- **Considers potential for delayed airway obstruction**

- Does not formulate appropriate management plan
- Fails to consider potential for delayed airway obstruction

The above framework is essentially how the selectors are instructed to evaluate candidates. It will vary for different scenarios, but the structure remains the same.

3.4 Questions and answers

<u>Scenario 1</u>: *Airway Emergency*

You are on call at 8pm on a Friday night. You are phoned by the local A&E department who would like you to urgently assess a 55 year old man with stridor in their resuscitation bay. You are told that he has been progressively having problems with breathing over the last 2 months and that his wife has now forced him to come into hospital. He is now breathless, tachypnoeic and very stridulous. He is a heavy smoker and has a history of alcohol abuse. Outline your management of this patient.

Answer 1

This is potentially an airway emergency and requires immediate review. I would tell the A&E doctor that I am on my way and I would ask them to inform an anaesthetist and ask for them to tell theatres that we need emergency airway and tracheostomy sets with appropriate tracheostomy tubes ready in the resuscitation area. I would advise them to get heliox for the patient but that if that were not present, supplemental oxygen via nasal specs would be required at least. Adrenaline nebs and dexamethasone should also be given. IV access and a full set of bloods, including group and save should be performed whilst ensuring that the anaesthetic team is called.

I would phone the on call consultant to inform them of the patient and to warn them that I might need their assistance.

On arrival I would assess the patient in an ALS ABC pattern whilst checking their observations and confirming their history. This should include allergies, medications, past medical history, last oral intake, events leading up to presenting problem (an AMPLE history). I would ask about weight loss and malaise.

My concerns with this patients history of smoking and alcohol use is that a malignancy may be causing airway obstruction.

If safe to do so I would carry out assessment of the airway via flexible laryngoscopy, examine the neck for lymphadenopathy and listen to the chest.

On examination via flexible laryngoscopy you find a large obstructing lesion arising from the left hypopharynx. What would you do now?

This patient may require an emergency tracheostomy and I would phone the consultant to update them on the situation and ask them to attend.

I would inform the patient and the relatives that there is swelling that is blocking the airway and that a tracheostomy may be required if he does not respond to the steroids and adrenaline. I would explain what this involves and say that we would hope it would only be a temporary measure. I would explain the procedure and ask the patient to consent if able to do so.

If the patient becomes stable I would ask for them to be transferred to a high dependency environment whilst preparations for CT scan are made. I would stay with the patient and be prepared to do an emergency tracheostomy if required.

If the patient failed to improve I would perform a local anaesthetic tracheostomy in theatres. If the patient could not make it to theatres or arrested I would perform an emergency tracheostomy. This should be a MDT decision between you and your Consultant A&E team and the anaesthetist Consultant.

Be prepared to explain how you would perform a local anaesthetic tracheostomy or an emergency tracheostomy.

Scenario 2: *Foreign body in the aerodigestive tract*

You are asked to see an 80-year-old gentleman who has come to A&E with a sore throat and difficulty swallowing since eating chicken for dinner last night. He has had a lateral soft tissue radiograph performed (Figure 3.1 is on your preparation sheet). Discuss your management of this patient.

Answer 2

This case may involve an airway foreign body and thus requires urgent assessment. I would attend the A&E department and assess the patient using the ALS ABC algorithm. Whilst doing this I would take an AMPLE history and note their observations. I would confirm the history and examine the patient's oral cavity and oropharynx. I would examine the neck for signs of surgical emphysema and I would ask for a flexible nasendoscope. I would also review the patient's radiology results.

He has had a lateral soft tissue radiograph (figure 3.1) which demonstrates opacity at the level of the arytenoid cartilage. Given his history of sudden onset after eating chicken this could be a chicken bone. There are no radiographic signs of surgical emphysema. A foreign body in this location requires urgent management not only because of pain and discomfort but also because severe swelling can occur in the aerodigestive tract (Figure 3.2), leading to compromise of the airway.

Figure 3.1 A foreign body in the aerodigestive tract

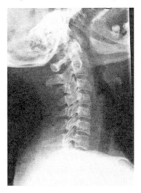

Figure 3.2 Increase in prevertebral soft tissue may be due to foreign body in aerodigestive tract

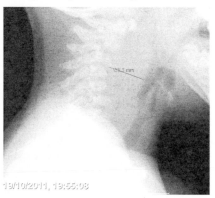

If the patient is stable I would confirm the location of the foreign body by flexible nasendoscopy.

Flexible nasendoscopy confirms the presence of a chicken bone just above the arytenoid cartilages.

Safe removal of the foreign body will require a general anaesthetic and direct pharyngo-laryngoscopy.

I would phone my consultant to inform them that I planned to take this patient to theatre and contact the theatres team and on call anaesthetist. I would explain the procedure to the patient (rigid pharyngo-laryngoscopy) and get informed consent to proceed.

Describe how you would perform direct pharyngoscopy and laryngoscopy

I would ensure all the required surgical equipment was available and that it was working. I would ask the anaesthetist if they were happy to use a microlaryngoscopy tube. I would position the patient with a small pillow under their shoulders and place a mouth guard to cover the teeth if appropriate. I would lubricate a rigid laryngoscope and ensure that the light was working. I would advance the scope using the ET tube as a guide and visualise the foreign body. I would then use forceps in my other hand to grab the foreign body and safely remove it with or in the scope. I would then use the scope to fully inspect the entire larynx, pharynx, tongue base and tonsillar fossae to confirm that there were no other foreign bodies and no signs of mucosal damage. If there was a suspicion of oesophageal/pharyngeal trauma I would pass an NGT.

After the procedure, if no NGT was passed, I would keep the patient nil by mouth for 4 hours and then to have a trial of sterile water with reassessment for any pain or discomfort on swallowing which might indicate a perforation. If there were no problems after a further 2 hours the patient could be started on soft diet. However, if I had passed an NGT, I would consider gastrograffin study the following day to rule out a perforation, especially if the patient is symptomatic with pain, surgical emphysema, tachycardia and reduced blood pressure.

<u>Scenario 3</u>: *Post-op haemorrhage (shock)*

You are the registrar on call. A nurse from the paediatric ward calls you to review a 3-year-old child who is unwell following a tonsillectomy that morning. She is not eating or drinking, is pale and her heart rate is going up. Discuss your management of this patient.

Answer 3

This child may be having a post-tonsillectomy bleed and as such management of this is an emergency and requires urgent action.

I would inform the nurse that I would be coming directly in to see the child. If I had an SHO on site I would contact them or the paediatrics team and ask them to attend the child and start resuscitation whilst I was on my way in. I would also ask them to contact the on call theatre team and let them know that we might need to take this child to theatre and that a Consultant Paediatric anaesthetist will be required.

On arrival I would assess the child using APLS guidelines via an ABC approach. I would take an AMPLE history from the child, parents and nurses.

If the child will tolerate it, I would carefully examine the mouth looking for clots or active bleeding in the tonsillar fossae.

There is active bleeding coming from the left tonsillar fossa at the inferior pole, what will you do?

This patient needs to be resuscitated and go to theatre for arrest of the tonsillar haemorrhage. I would ask the SHO/Paeds to take a cross match sample for 2 units if one has not already been taken.

Remember to revise your paediatric resuscitation guidelines for calculating bolus and maintenance fluids as well as weight estimation (Table 3.2).

Table 3.2 Paediatric Resuscitation Guidelines

Paediatric weight estimation	(Age x2) +4 = e.g. for 3 year old (3x2) +4= 10kg
Circulating blood volume of a child	85ml/kg e.g. for 3 year old = 850ml
Fluid challenge	20mls/kg normal saline is generally safe
Maintenance fluid	4mls/kg/hr for the first 10kg 2mls/kg/hr for the second 10kg 1ml/kg/hr for each additional kg e.g. 24kg child (4x10 + 2x10 + 4) = 64mls/hr

I would discuss management with the theatre team, paediatric team, anaesthetic team and my consultant and recommend that the patient requires surgical arrest of the haemorrhage.

I would speak to the parents and explain to them that this is a serious problem and that management of this requires a general anaesthetic and stopping the bleeding in the operating theatre. I would explain that we may need to give a blood transfusion and I would obtain informed consent for the procedure.

The parents are Jehovah's witnesses and refuse the blood transfusion.

I would explain again that this is a serious situation and that their child is already showing signs of shock from blood loss. There is potential for cardiac arrest and death from blood loss. I would stress the need to go to theatre and that we would use other forms of resuscitation fluid if possible. I would contact the consultant to explain about this issue.

If there was time and it was felt to be required a petition could be made to a high court judge for treatment of a child under 16 against the wishes of the parent. If this would cause unacceptable delay the child could be treated against the wishes of the parents with judicial approval sought afterwards.

The child is anaesthetised in theatre; explain what procedure you would perform.

I would use a headlight and use suction to remove all the blood from the mouth and oropharynx. I would gently remove any clots in the tonsillar fossa and identify the bleeding point. If possible I would try and use ties or bipolar diathermy to arrest the bleeding. I would also consider the use of adrenaline soaked swabs to aid with haemostasis whilst performing this. If this failed I would pack the fossa with Surgicel™ and tie the tonsillar pillars together with a stitch. I would then use a nasogastric tube to suction clear any swallowed blood from the stomach. Following that, I would wait to ensure haemostasis and arrange for the child to have monitoring and review post operatively. I would then return to the ward and speak with the parents about the outcome of the procedure. Finally, I would ensure that a record of the procedure was kept for the monthly morbidity and mortality discussion and inform my consultant of the outcome if competent to perform the procedure with minimal supervision.

Scenario 4: *Post – operative orbital swelling*

You have finished your morning operating list and at 1pm you are called by one of the nurses in recovery who would like you to see a patient. He is a 48 year old man who underwent a FESS polypectomy at 11 am this morning. The operating was uneventful but he has now developed right sided orbital swelling, diplopia and is bleeding from both nostrils. Discuss your management of this patient.

Answer 4

This is an emergency as there is risk to vision.

I would attend the patient and make a quick assessment of ABC based on the ALS protocol. I would start any resuscitation required based on my findings.

I would take a focussed history on the when the swelling started, whether they had any symptoms such as diplopia or restricted eye movement or any change to their visual acuity or colour perception. I would ask how long the epistaxis has been going on for and whether the patient had any risk factors for bleeding (anticoagulant medications, coagulopathy etc). I would check whether they had eaten since the operations and confirm their allergies and other medical history.

I would ask for the notes and start examining the patient. I would assess them for signs of optic nerve compression firstly starting with colour vision assessment. You can get an Ishihara chart for your Smart phone which I would use or I would test the patient on coloured objects nearby. I would check their visual acuity by asking them to read something (an ID badge for example). I would then check eye movements and ask the patient if they could see double at any stage that would very likely indicate ocular muscle restriction. I would also assess the degree of epistaxis and determine whether this needed urgent action (i.e. packing).

If there were signs of optic nerve compression I would have about 1 hour from the onset of compression to save vision. If these signs were present at this stage I would phone the consultant, contact theatres, keep the patient nil by mouth and consent them for returning to theatre.

If access to theatre was going to be delayed I would consider performing a lateral canthotomy on the ward under local anaesthetic as this would help to release pressure in the orbit and buy time for going to theatre.

Lateral canthotomy:

1-2 mls of 2%lignocaine with 1:80000 adrenaline

Clip with artery forceps towards orbital rim

Cut laterally down to orbital rim (DO NOT damage conjunctiva)

Pull lower lid down with forceps, visualise inferior lateral canthal tendon and divide (globe and fat will prolapse)

Re-suture in 24-48 hours

Scenario 5: *Post-operative facial nerve palsy*

You are about to leave the hospital at the end of a busy list when one of the patients asks you to review a patient from one of the other teams list. Mrs X is a 55 year old lady who had a left combined approach tympanoplasty 2 hours ago. She is now complaining of weakness of the left side of her face and can't close her eyelid. Discuss your management of this patient

Answer 5

This patient has a post operative facial nerve weakness which requires urgent assessment.

I would attend the patient and make a quick assessment of their ABCs (as per ALS guidelines) and check their observations. I would take a history from the patient regarding when this problem started (immediately that they came round from the anaesthetic or subsequently) and I would ask if the nurse could get a hold of the notes so that I could review the operation note. I would review exactly what was carried out during the procedure paying particular note to any mention of local anaesthetic used and whether the facial nerve was approached at all. I would quickly cover the patients past medical history, medications and allergies taking note of any previous history of facial nerve paralysis

I would move on to assess the facial nerve function and to firstly determine whether this is an upper or lower motor neuron problem (forehead sparing in UMN) and to grade the severity of palsy using the House-Brackmann score *(learn this)*. If there is a head bandage on I would carefully take this down and assess whether there was any swelling below the skin incision suggestive of haematoma. I would not remove any packing.

The potential causes of the facial nerve palsy are the effect of any local anaesthetic used or a result of direct trauma to the nerve or compression from post-operative bleeding or oedema. I would phone the consultant who had performed the operation and ask for their advice as if they were confident that the nerve was not likely to have been damaged then the patient could undergo a period of observation for several hours to see if the local anaesthetic might wear off. If it was felt that the nerve was at risk then the consultant would likely opt to take the patient back to theatre for exploration.

Scenario 6: *Acute mastoiditis*

You are asked by your FY2 to see a 3 year old child who has attended A&E with right sided pain and swelling behind the ear (Figure 3.3) as well fever, right sided headache and malaise. Discuss your approach to the management of this patient.

Figure 3.3 Clinical photograph of a painful fluctuant swelling behind the right ear

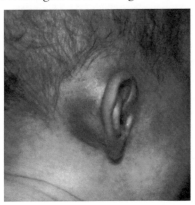

Answer 6

This patient potentially has acute mastoiditis and has symptoms of sepsis or meningitis so urgent assessment is required.

I would attend the patient and carry out initial assessment by and ALS ABC approach. I would start any necessary resuscitation and take blood samples for culture, full blood count, U&Es, LFTs and group & save. I would take a full history focussing on previous ear infections or surgery and to clarify what symptoms they were having. I would ask about past medical history, regular medication, allergies and when they last ate. If they had a temperature I would start antibiotics based on local policy.

I would then move on to clinical examination. I would start by examining the ears focussing initially on the mastoid looking for swelling, erythema and signs of collection or abscess formation. I would then perform otoscopy looking for signs of active infection, cholesteatoma or otitis media. I would move on to examine all the cranial nerves, especially the facial nerve.

On examination you find that there is a fluctuant swelling behind the right ear but normal appearances of the tympanic membrane. The patient has weakness of their right 6th cranial nerve and is complaining of double vision on right lateral gaze. There is tenderness around the right eye but no erythema and the patient is complaining that it is painful when the light is shone in their eye. What are your concerns now?

This patient has signs of right sided acute mastoiditis as well as symptoms suggestive of meningitis and problems affecting the 5th and 6th cranial nerves. This would fit in with a diagnosis of Gradenigos syndrome *(bonus marks here for knowing this, not essential for the answer)*.

This patient would require urgent drainage of the mastoid infection via a cortical mastoidectomy. I would phone the consultant on call to ask for their help with this case. I would keep the patient nil by mouth, obtain informed consent for this procedure and inform theatres that this patient requires urgent surgery. If there were delays for proceeding to theatre (e.g. a case already on the table) I would consider requesting an urgent CT scan as long as this did not delay surgery. A drain would be left in postoperatively. I would discuss management of the meningitis with the paediatric and neurology team.

Scenario 7: *Peri-orbital cellulitis*

You are the on call registrar and whilst at home you receive a call from your A&E department asking for a review of a 15 year old boy has attended with their parents. He has developed a swelling around the left eye (Figure 3.4). What would be your approach to managing this patient?

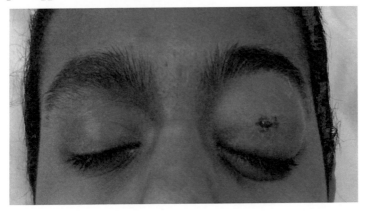

Figure 3.4 Clinical photograph showing left peri-orbital cellulitis

Answer 7

This patient potentially has peri-orbital cellulitis which can threaten the vision in the affected eye as well as potentially causing intra-cranial complications. As such I would want to assess this patient urgently and I would ask the A&E staff to insert a cannula, take bloods including cultures, resuscitate the teenager as required and start antibiotics as per local guidelines. I would ask them to keep the patient nil-by-mouth and contact the ENT SHO asking them to attend with a paediatric nasendoscope if available. I would also ask the A&E team to liaise with ophthalmology as they may be required to assess the patient vision. I would then attend the patient.

On arrival you go to assess the patient and his appearance is shown (Figure 3.4). How would continue to manage him?

The photograph shows erythema and swelling around the left eye that is consistent with peri-orbital cellulitis. I would be concerned that due to the degree of swelling there might an acute risk to vision. After introducing myself I would take a focussed history from teenager and the parents particularly asking whether there had been a recent upper respiratory tract infection or sinusitis. I would ask whether he had been taking oral antibiotics prior to coming in to hospital and at what time the swelling was first noticed. As this teenager may need an urgent operation I would take an AMPLE history asking about allergies, medications, past medical history, last oral intake and any other events leading up to the presentation.

I would then move on to examining the patient asking him to try to open his eye or to open his eye for him in order to assess his colour vision with an Ishihara chart and his visual acuity with a Snellen chart. If the patient will allow me I would like to examine his nose endoscopically to look for signs of acute sinusitis or infection.

The patient is unable to open his eye. How would you proceed?

I am unable to assess the vision adequately and I would be concerned that intra-orbital swelling could be compromising vision. Given that there is an imminent risk to vision I would want to prepare the patient for theatre for an external or endoscopic drainage of a peri-orbital collection after organising an urgent CT scan with contrast.

I am particularly interested in the CT axial images. I would discuss the patient with the on-call consultant and (depending on my competency) if they agree with my management plan I would ask them to attend for the procedure. I would explain to the parents the clinical findings and the potential risk to vision necessitating urgent surgery. I would explain to them the nature of the procedure, its goals and the potential complications of operating and of not operating. I would then check their understanding and prepare a consent form and ask them to sign it. I would reassure them and answer any questions. I would contact the emergency list anaesthetist and explain that this is an urgent case that should be done as soon as possible. I would contact the theatre team and ask them to prepare both a paediatric FESS set and a basic plastics set If it will not delay getting to theatre I would arrange a CT scan of the brain and sinuses to delineate the anatomy, classify the severity and help guide the procedure. I would make sure that the patient had been given IV antibiotics, nasal decongestants and suitable analgesia. I would also discuss the case with the paediatric and ophthalmology teams.

There is an emergency in the operating theatre at the moment and the radiologists agree to do an immediate CT scan (Figure 3.5). What can you see and do you know any scoring systems used for grading peri-orbital cellulitis?

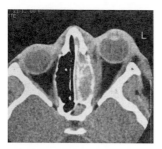

Figure 3.5 Axial CT scan showing a subperiosteal abscess involving the left eye

Based on the CT scan this patient may have a Chandler III or subperiosteal abscess (Table 3.3). There is proptosis of the right eye with a sub-periosteal abscess medially within the orbit. This is related to opacification within the right ethmoid air cells suggestive of sinusitis as the origin of the abscess.

Table 3.3 Chandler's grading for peri-orbital cellulitis

Grade I	Pre-septal cellulitis	This refers to inflammatory oedema anterior to tarsal plate of eyelid causing the eyelids to swell. This condition is caused due to restricted venous drainage. The eyelids though swollen are not tender. Since the inflammation doesn't involve postseptal structures there is no chemosis, Extraocular muscle movement limitations and vision impairment. Proptosis may be present to a mild degree.
Grade II	Orbital cellulitis	Orbital cellulitis causes marked oedema and inflammation of orbital contents without abscess formation. It is important to look for signs of proptosis and reduced ocular mobility as these are reliable signs of orbital cellulitis. Chemosis is usually present in this group.
Grade III	Sub-periosteal abscess	In this group abscess develops in the space between the bone and periosteum (hence subperiosteal abscess). Orbital contents may be displaced in an inferolateral direction due to the mass effect of

		accumulating pus. Chemosis and proptosis are usually present. Decreased ocular mobility and loss of vision is rare in this group
Grade IV	Orbital abscess	Orbital abscess involves collection of purulent material within the orbital contents. This could be caused due to relentless progression of orbital cellulitis or rupture of orbital abscess. Severe proptosis, complete ophthalmoplegia, and loss of vision are commonly seen in this group of patients.
Grade V	Cavernous sinus thrombosis	Here there is development of bilateral ocular signs is the classic feature of patients belonging to this group. These patients classically manifest with fever, headache, photophobia, proptosis, ophthalmoplegia and loss of vision. Cranial nerve palsies involving III, IV, V1, V2 and VI are common.

What operation is required for this patient?

There are two approaches for subperiosteal abscess drainage – open or endoscopic. An open approach involves a Lynch-Howarth incision down onto bone with the preiosteum of the medial orbit being raised to gain access to and to drain the sub-periosteal abscess. A drain can be left in place to be removed at a later stage.

An endoscopic approach would involve adequately preparing the nose with a decongestant such as Moffett's solution or adrenaline soak patties and performing a targeted FESS aiming to open the ethmoid air cells and opening the lamina to drain the abscess medially. I would ask my consultant as to which method they prefer and to ask for them to supervise and assist me if possible.

Post-operatively I would ensure that the patient was on IV antibiotics, nasal decongestants and was having regular eye observations. If they have not attended already I would ask for an ophthalmology consultation. I would speak to the parents to let them know how the procedure has gone and what the plan is for their continuing care.

Tips:

- Revise your ALS, ATLS and APLS guidelines. Knowing these algorithms and following them is essential.

- Talk to your registrars or colleagues. Ask them about specific emergencies they have dealt with as a "real world answer" will show the interviewers that you are aware of the practical issues with management of these problems.

- Get your seniors to grill you on how you would manage these problems. This may help to correct any misunderstandings you have as well as getting you used to answering these questions.

- Talk to your consultants – what would they expect you to do if you were the registrar on call.

3.5 Marking scheme

In 2012, a total of 25 marks are allocated for the management of a clinical scenario (peri-orbital cellulitis). Marks were awarded for recognising the urgency of the case, highlighting salient aspects of the history, examination, appropriate investigation, relevant classification, team approach and treatment (medical and surgical). Nearly 25 percent of the marks were set aside for knowledge of appropriate examination of the nose (anterior rhinoscopy and nasendoscopy) and eyes (colour vision, visual acuity, eye movements and papillary reflexes). Four marks were allocated for the global assessments of your clinical management skills.

Chapter 4

Communication Station

4.1 Overview

The teaching of communication skills has become increasingly popular over the past ten years and a communication assessment is now seen in almost every SpR interview. Though candidates may be effective communicators at work, it does not necessarily translate that they will score highly in this part of the interview. Good candidates throw away easy marks by missing key phrases and actions that the interviewer is looking for or may find it difficult to display their natural effective communication style in an environment that is unnatural, stressful and often involves communicating with an actor. It is therefore essential that you practice your communication skills and use them at the interview.

Communication skills stations in the interview setting are task based. You will be provided with a specific task that will involve a simulated encounter with a patient or relative over a 10-15 minute period. There will usually be two interviewers marking the station and sometimes a third person who may be a lay representative that will give their opinion on your communication style. The best way to approach the communication station is to break it up into manageable stages. In this chapter we highlight the four stages of communication.

4.2 Four stages of communication

Stage 1: *The information sheet*

From the start you will be given a printed information sheet explaining the communication scenario. Sometimes there is an allocation of a separate five minute period to read through it or you may be asked to read it and then start the scenario when you're ready. It is essential that you keep calm and absorb the information accurately. It is all too easy to let nerves and time pressure get the better of you and launch into the consultation without fully understanding what information you are supposed to be discussing.

The first piece of information you should filter is what type of scenario you are going to be faced with. Common scenarios are listed below and you should prepare an approach for each of them.

- **Information giving**
    - Explaining a result
    - Explaining a procedure / consent
    - Explaining a problem or mistake
    - Dealing with a complaint
    - Breaking bad news

- **Information gathering**
    - Taking a history

The second piece of information you should try and glean is what type of patient you are likely to face. This will depend on the clinical scenario and should direct your communication style.

- The angry patient: Simulated patients often adopt an angry communication style when there has been a delay or mistake in the patient or relatives management. You might also meet the angry patient in a breaking bad news situation especially when discussing it with a relative. The actor should be allowed to vent their anger by using good active listening skills on your part. Use non-confrontational body language such as outstretched palms. Do not be afraid to apologise to the patient or relative. The patient is usually angry as they feel their needs and concerns have not been addressed properly or they have been overlooked. To compensate for this make sure you verbalise how important you take their concerns and how determined you are to sort them out. Do not under any circumstances be confrontational.

- The upset/distressed patient: If the scenario revolves around breaking bad news, the patient will clearly be upset. It is therefore important to modify your communication and adopt a sensitive and empathetic approach.

- The concerned or worried patient/relative: If the scenario involves explaining treatment to a relative or explaining a normal investigation result the actor is likely to adopt an anxious role. The key is to provide as much support as possible and provide plenty of opportunities for the actor to ask questions. It is also important to check they understand the information provided.

In some cases the type of patient will not be obvious. Do not worry, just allow the conversation to flow naturally.

Stage 2: *The introduction*

A strong introduction is key and will help win round both the interviewers and actor. You should make up and practice your own introduction and include the following points.

- Greeting

- Checking the patients identity

- Check if they have anybody they would like to join them

- Introducing yourself and your role and position

- Explain why you're meeting

- Checking what they know so far

Stage 3: *Communication*

This is the main part of the assessment. Marks will be allocated on your verbal communication skills, non-verbal communication skills and accuracy of information.

Verbal communication skills

- Active listening: Active listening (Figure 4.10 is simply demonstrating that you are listening to the patient. This can be through non-verbal and verbal communication. Verbal active listening skills can involve single words of acknowledgement expressed whilst the patient is speaking. Summarising is a useful verbal active listening technique. After a patient has finished talking summarise what they have just said to acknowledge you have listened and understood what they have said before giving an answer.

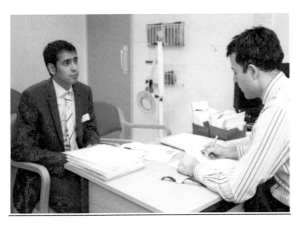

Figure 4.1   Active listening is an important part of communication (Mr Chatrath on ENTTZAR Event 2011)

- Empathy: Marks are often allocated for demonstrating empathy during the communication assessment at interview. Whilst many people might feel empathetic we do not always express it, especially when communicating with an actor where the medical problem is fictional. It is therefore important to make a conscious effort to demonstrate empathy during the communication assessment. The best way to achieve this is to acknowledge and express the emotions and feelings of the patient. For instance if the simulated patient is upset you should state "I can see you are very upset and that is understandable" or if you are delivering complex information "I appreciate that this is a lot of information to take in and it might be confusing". In bad news situations avoid using phrases like "I know this must be really difficult for you" or similar as often you have never been directly in that situation yourself. Instead try "I can only imagine how difficult this is" or something similar. It is also a good idea to explore the simulated patient's emotions during the consultation by trying to fit in phrases such as "and how did that make you feel?"

- Sign posting: When explaining information to patients it is often useful to sign post. This refers to dividing the information into categories and explaining each category in turn. For example if explaining a surgical procedure you could try.

  "What I suggest we do is: I discuss the procedure itself, what happens afterwards and also the risks and benefits and then give you a chance at the end to ask questions. Is that OK with you?"….."Good, so firstly the procedure itself……", "secondly, after the procedure…."etc.

  Signposting will give your explanation clarity and allow the patient to refer back to a particular point should they not understand something.

- Checking for understanding & questions: When ever you deliver information you should always make a point of pausing at certain points to check they understand you and give a number of opportunities to ask questions. It is also important to avoid medical jargon, however if medical terms are used do give an explanation of the term directly afterwards.

Open and closed questions: Try and keep your questions open and general and allow the patient to volunteer details themselves. Avoid firing direct questions in rapid succession.

Non-verbal communication skills

- Sitting position: You should sit in a comfortable position without slouching and ensuring your hands are not crossed. You should sit near the patient and ideally not facing directly to them as this can appear threatening. Avoid having barriers in the way such as a desk.

- Eye contact: You should use appropriate eye contact. This means not trying to stare constantly at the patient but also ensuring you make frequent eye contact especially when greeting and disengaging.

- Active listening: When the actor is talking you should appear interested, maintain eye contact and use body language to indicate you are listening to what they are saying. This can include nodding your head in agreement and the use of appropriate facial expression to mirror what the patient is explaining to you. It is important that the interviewer sees you are engaging in active listening but it is also important not to over do it and appear unnatural. The best way of achieving this balance is through practice or reflecting on how you best communicate with patients at work.

- Empathy: Ensure that your expressions and tone roughly mirror that of the actor. An obvious example would be to avoid smiling and appear serious/sombre in breaking bad news scenarios. If the simulated patient becomes upset during the assessment there is usually a box of tissues near by. By offering a tissue you are demonstrating you recognise the patient is upset and are trying to comfort them.

- Silence: The use of silence is an excellent non-verbal communication skill. After a patient has finished explaining something wait before giving your response. This allows the patient time to continue talking if they wish to do so and makes your response appear more thought out.

Accuracy of information

- You must ensure the information you deliver to the simulated patient is accurate. If you are unsure about something do not try and guess it but instead explain you will ask your consultant or find out the answer and get back to them.

Breaking bad news

Breaking bad news requires a specific communication style that can be broken down into stages which you should prepare in your head before starting.

1. Explore what the patient already knows their main concerns.

2. Set out a plan for discussion and offer the chance to ask questions.

3. Start to explain the result checking for understanding as you go.

4. Before delivering the bad news use warning shots (warn, **W**) and pause (**P**) to prepare the patient.

5. After delivering the bad news pause and check (**C**) the patient wants you to continue and allow the simulated patient to respond

6. Be supportive and explore concerns and feelings after breaking bad news

7. Answer questions and form plan for the future

8. Close with contact points and further support such as a nurse or relative

Stage 4: *Closure*

Bringing the consultation to a close should involve the following

- Opportunity to ask any further questions

- Opportunity to re-explain a point discussed

- Summarise the discussion

- Form an action plan for the future

- Provide contact details for how the patient can reach you should they need to

- If the patient is upset or anxious ask if they would like you to call someone or offer them the support of a nurse.

Knowing when to finish can be difficult in the communication station. There is usually a warning that there are only two minutes left signalled by a bell or knock on the door. You should not ignore this information and should prepare to close the consultation if you hear it. Sometimes you will get to a stage where you feel you've come to the end of the consultation even though you have time left. In this case ask the actor "is there anything else I'm missing" and "is there anything else you'd like me to discuss or go over again". If the answer is no to both then you can safely close knowing you're likely to have covered all of the points.

4.3 Communication skills courses

A good way to prepare for the communication assessment at interview is to attend a general communication skills course and a specific ENT mock interview course. Whilst there are currently very few specific courses on communication skills for medical interviews, there are numerous communication skills courses to help people through their membership exams. Communication assessment for membership examinations are practically the same as communication assessments in interview and therefore a lot can be gained from attending these courses. Events offering mock interviews in communication skills are also invaluable (Figure 4.2).

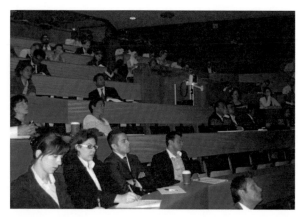

Figure 4.2 Delegates on ENTTZAR ST3 mock interview course 2011

4.4 Body Language relevant to effective communication

Most candidates will spend time sharpening their clinical and management knowledge and buying expensive new interview outfits; however, few prepare for arguably one of the most important components when presenting yourself to others - your body language. Albert Mehrabian, Professor Emeritus of Psychology, UCLA, is credited with the 7%-38%-55% rule of human communication. Despite his original studies being regarding communication of positive and negative feelings and attitudes in women they are widely (mis)interpreted as the '3 Vs' for verbal, vocal and visual communication. That is when a person is communicating, words account for 7%, tone of voice 38% and body language for 58% of liking.

Do and Don'ts

- The first impression is vital and many people make their mind up about a person in the first few moments of meeting them. Despite interviewers consciously trying not to do this, sub-consciously an impression is still made.

- Smiling is essential. It is difficult not to like someone who has a nice smile (Figure 4.3).

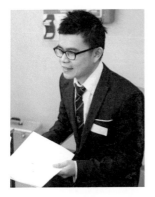

Figure 4.3 Smiling is a vital component of non-verbal communication

- It is vital to dress correctly and appropriately. Dressing sombrely with a clean appearance is a form of echoing, your interviewers certainly will be appropriately dressed and this will work to your advantage.

• Sit with a comfortable open posture as this will impart a relaxed, open attitude. Sitting with both arms and legs crossed with a closed posture does suggest a defensive, negative attitude. Aligning yourself towards your interviewer by leaning slightly forward projects interest and engages you with the situation.

• Postural echoing occurs when people share the same views, the same status or like each other (Figure 4.4). A good example of this, is when sitting with a friend at a bar, drinking from your glass at the same time often happens without conscious effort. This is postural echoing and implies that your thinking, behaviour and outlook are similar.

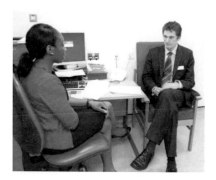

Figure 4.4 An example of postural echoing during an interview on ENTTZAR ST3 course.

• During the interview it is vital to be subtle about this.

• Paraphrasing is another useful technique when asked a question, verbal mirroring indicates that you have understood and have been listening; however overdoing this will have the opposite effect.

- Naturally when meeting new groups, we also find people that look at us directly and smile to be more likeable and attractive. If you're liked, you're more likely to be successful.

- Other top tips for success are to walk in confidently, do not adjust your tie or skirt, do this outside. Say hello to everyone as they are introduced to you, smile and make eye contact, if a handshake is offered make sure that yours is firm.

- Find a comfortable position to sit, without rocking or shaking your leg or foot. Don't cross your arms or drum your fingers - this gives an impression of being unable to focus and can be very distracting.

- Fidgeting also always looks bad, in particular touching your nose and head is said to suggest dishonesty.

- Speak clearly addressing both interviewers with good volume and not too fast, be measured. Keep your responses succinct, usually a two sentence answer is appropriate, don't ramble on. Don't hyperventilate, keep your breathing regular and calm, any signs of stress and you could be quizzed further.

- Use head nodding and postural echoing in moderation and with subtlety.

- Your interviewers will have a keen sense of smell, don't ruin things by smelling like a tobacconist, brewery or perfumery!

- Remember, it is widely accepted that non verbal behaviour correlates statistically significantly with interview success.

- This is an area where everyone can improve their performance by practice, there is also professional help available from body language and specialist interview coaches.

Top tip: Remember, it is widely accepted that non-verbal behaviour correlates statistically significantly with interview success.

4.5 Questions and Answers

Here we present five typical cases which may be suitable for communication skills. Because of the complex verbal and non-verbal interactions involve in communication, it is difficult to provide perfect model answers. Therefore, we have opted to present the scenarios and key points in a table format (Table 4.1).

Table 4.1 Examples of scenarios that may be used in the communication skills station

	Scenarios	Key areas where marks are likely to be allocated
1	A 45 year old roofer with moderate hearing loss in his right ear due to otosclerosis. His left ear is normal.	Discussion of pathology Treatment options Implications of vertigo in a roofer
	He is keen on surgery (sister had good results from similar op) but is only bread winner for	Percentage risk of dead ear, no improvement, worse hearing.

	large family of six.	Empathy
2	A 46 year old female with difficulty swallowing, ear ache (especially when swallowing) wt loss, long history of iron deficiency anaemia, non smoker and non-drinker. Investigations reveals T4 post cricoid carcinoma	Recognising post-cricoid cancer is one of the very few cancers not linked to smoking and drinking Breaking bad news (**WPC** method, see earlier text) Counselling with regards to a big operation: voice box, top of oesophagus, and neck nodes removed How will she eat? NGT/PEG? Alternative and additional treatment (RT) Complications and long term outcomes? Empathy as patient feel hard-done-by because only smokers and drinkers should get head and neck cancers
3	A 14 year old boy who has been having nose bleeds.	Anaemic Unilateral haemorrhagic nasal mass Dangerous to biopsy because of bleeding (due to lack of contractile tissue in blood vessels but normal clotting) CT shows bowing of

		posterior maxillary wall, MRI shows tumour consistent with juvenile angiofribroma.
		Treatment options
		Recurrence if basisphenoid regions is not removed
		Potentially disfiguring surgery needed Patient wants to be an actor like his dad
		Empathy
4	A 25 year old male student who fell over whilst drunk. Sustained temporal bone fracture and right dead ear. His ambition is to join the Navy	Discuss CT findings of temporal bone fracture.
		Explain audiological results suggesting a right dead ear
		Discuss inability to join navy (or any uniform jobs) due to SSD
		Discuss role of cross aid and BAHA
		Counsel regarding protection of other ear (no party, no alcohol, no motorcycle, no noisy environment)
		Empathy
5	A 40 year old chef who	Anosmia secondary to

complains of inability to taste the food he is cooking. MRI shows brain tumour (olfactory neuroblastoma).	olfactory neuroblastoma
	Has to give up job
	Need to change gas to electric cooker
	Need for smoke alarm
	Importance of noting sell by dates on food,
	Empathy

4.6 Marking scheme

In 2012, a total of 25 marks are allocated for communication station. The scenario involved communicating with the son of a patient who had an airway obstruction. Marks were given for introducing yourself, establishing a rapport, discussing the problem without using jargon, honesty, verbal, non-verbal, fluency and empathy. Discussion surrounding a possible tracheostomy was also included and awarded 4 points. Global rating of communication skills accounted for 8 marks!

Chapter 5

Clinical Skills Station

5.1 Overview

The clinical skills station is designed to test hand eye co-ordination, practical clinical skills and/or interpretation of diagnostic information. In 2011, the candidate had to draw and label a tympanic membrane, setting up a microscope and inserting a grommet on a model. In previous years of SpR interviews in the London Deanery, this station had tested flexible nasendoscopy, direct laryngoscopy, tonsil ties, instrument suturing and hand ties. In general it is always important that you introduce yourself, stay calm, convey the message that you've done this before, talk through what you are doing, naming items, while saying what you'd do in clinical practice.

Surprisingly, in 2012 the clinical skills station assessed the candidate's ability to perform tuning fork tests and interpreting audiograms. In this chapter we will present some tips on the practical procedures that are likely to appear in the ST3 interview, including some tips on the interpretation of audiograms and tuning fork tests. In this chapter we present the essential information on skills you are likely to be tested on at the national selection process, including flexible nasendoscopy, rigid endoscopy, microlaryngoscopy, sutures and suturing and types of needles. We also provide a brief account of clinical audiology, audiograms and masking, with some relevant questions and answers.

5.2 Flexible nasendoscopy

Nasal endoscopy is commonly used in the evaluation of the nasal and sinus passages in the ENT out-patient setting.

The equipment used is based on the rods lens system invented by Harold Horace Hopkins (1918-1994) and was introduced to the field of otolaryngology by Karl Storz (1911-1996). It provides a high-quality, direct magnified view of the examining area and facilitates in the evaluation of the nasal mucosa and sinonasal anatomy. It plays an important role in identifying pathology and monitoring treatment, both medical and/or surgical.

There are two forms of nasal endoscopes available; the flexible fibre-optic endoscope (Figure 5.1) and the rigid endoscope. The flexible endoscopes have the advantage of being manipulated in multiple directions, providing views as far as the hypopharynx; the rigid endoscope is limited to the post-nasal space.

The rigid endoscopes are available in diameters of 1.0 – 4.0mm and have tips of varying angles (usually 0°-70°). The different angled endoscopes allow the clinician to visualize various areas within the nasal cavity and sinuses. The advantages of rigid endoscopy are:

- Aid in obtaining tissue samples
- Better control of epistaxis
- Provides the ability to perform surgery

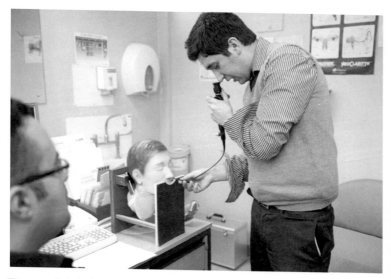

Figure 5.1 A ST3 candidate performing FNE on a manikin

Indications

Nasal endoscopy should be seen as a vital tool for evaluating a patient with sinonasal symptoms, without which the examination is incomplete. Nasal pathology can be missed in up to 40% of patients in whom only anterior rhinoscopy is performed.

There are numerous clinical indicators for performing nasal endoscopy and include:

- Initial evaluation of patients with sinonasal symptoms (e.g. head and facial pain, chronic nasal catarrh, nasal obstruction/congestion or anosmia)
- Management of epistaxis
- Monitoring response to treatment or recurrence of pathology after FESS
- Evaluating unilateral nasal disease

- Obtaining biopsies of nasal masses, lesions or mucopurulent secretions
- Removal of foreign bodies
- Evaluating the nasopharynx for lymphoid hyperplasia or Eustachian tube abnormalities
- Evaluation of suspected or known cerebrospinal fluid (CSF) rhinorrhea
- Evaluating epiphora
- Evaluating pharyngitis and laryngitis
- Assessing a hoarse voice
- Evaluating hypopharyngeal disease

Contraindications

There are no absolute contraindications for nasal endoscopy; however, you should be aware of patients that are at increased risk of complications. Nasal endoscopy should be performed cautiously in patients with bleeding tendencies (e.g. on anticoagulants) so as not to cause epistaxis. There is also the risk of a vasovagal episode in an anxious individual or in a patient with cardiovascular disease.

Recording Evaluation

During the examination it is important to record the findings accurately and in a systematic order. The Table 5.1 below shows some of the items to record in the nasal cavity.

Table 5.1 Documentation of Flexible Nasendoscopy

Mucosal Surface	Moist, Dry, Telangiectasa, Crusting, Perforation
Mucosal Colour	Pink, Hyperaemic, Pale
Pus	Identify presence/absence and location
Secretions	Viscous, Thin, Bloodstained
Turbinates	Swollen, Absent, Adhesions
Anatomical Variations	Septal deviations, Spurs, Concha Bullosa, Accessory ostia, Evidence of previous surgery

Procedure

As with all procedures, nasal endoscopy has 3 separate components; pre-procedural steps, the procedure itself and, post-procedural care.

Pre-procedural steps

Verbal consent should be carried out ensuring the patient is adequately prepared as this may be a first time experience for many. Warn the patient of potential complications: sneezing, coughing, gagging, "tearing" from the eyes and bleeding.

The procedure is usually carried out without premedication. If the nasal mucosa is sensitive or very swollen then a 0.5% phenylephrine and 5% lidocaine spray can be used to decongest and anaesthetize the area respectively. Ensure you have checked for allergies and allow 5 minutes if used. The patient should be sat upright against a chair, so as to prevent them from leaning away.

Equipment

Determine if you are going to perform either flexible or rigid endoscopy. The flexible endoscope is usually available only as one size in most centers. If performing rigid endoscopy, the 0° wide-angled scope (4mm) is the standard scope for nasal endoscopy, however, a 30° scope is beneficial as described in the section on technique. Smaller diameter scopes (2.7mm, 1mm) should be used if access is limited, for example in septal deviation or in small children. Other equipment that will be required:

- Tissue for patient to wipe tears and nose
- Lubricating gel
- Antifog solution (an alcohol street can be used alternatively)
- Microbiology swabs
- Light source +/- monitor
- Sinonasal instruments – Freer's elevator, through cutting instrument

Technique

The endoscopic examination should follow a systematic approach ensuring all areas are evaluated. Tips for aiding visualization of the larynx and hypopharynx are given in Table 5.2. The steps for flexible nasoendoscopy can be considered as follows:

- Perform anterior rhinoscopy to determine through which nasal cavity you will proceed
- Advance the scope along the inferior nasal cavity to the post-nasal space and assess for lymphoid hyperplasia
- Examine eustachian tube orifices, fossae of Rosenmuller and posterior pharyngeal wall
- Ask patient to swallow and breathe through nose to help advance scope towards hypopharynx

- Examine posterior aspects of tonsils, tongue base, epiglottis and valeculla
- Advance further to laryngopharynx
- Examine piriform fossae, false vocal cords, true vocal cords, arytenoid cartilages, anterior and posterior commisures and ventricles
- Can be possible to see causes of subglottic stenosis in some cases
- Assess vocal cord movements by asking to patient to say "eee" or "count from 1 to 10"
- On withdrawing the scope examine the nasal passageway including the inferior and middle turbinates
- Repeat the same on the other side if possible as far as the post-nasal space

Table 5.2 Tips to aid visualization during flexible nasendoscopy

Useful manoeuvres during flexible nasendoscopy
Extend chin to open airway
Turning the patients head to left/right will open up right/left piriform fossa, respectively.
Sticking out tongue to assess tongue base and vallecullae
Performing valsalva to open up ventricles

5.3 Rigid endoscopy

As previously mentioned, a 4mm 0° is usually selected first and three separate passes of the scope in to each nasal cavity are made. With each pass the appearance of the nasal mucosa and nasal cavity structures is examined.

First Pass

The patients head is kept slightly flexed and the $0°$ scope passed towards the nasopharynx whilst visualizing the nasal floor. The inferior turbinate and inferior meatus (opening of nasolacrimal duct) is examined. The scope is advanced further posterior to the nasopharynx where the Eustachian tube orifices, fossa of Rosenmüller, soft palate motility and posterior pharyngeal wall inspected. In children the adenoids should be evaluated also.

Second Pass

The $0°$ scope is passed between the middle and inferior turbinates. This is to examine the middle meatus, fontanelles and to assess for accessory maxillary ostia. A freer's elevator can be used to gently medialise the middle turbinate in order to visualize the middle meatus. The scope should then be passed medially and posterior to the middle turbinate in order to examine the sphenoethmoidal recess which is located medial to the middle and superior turbinates. The ethmoid bulla, infundibulum and uncinate process are examined by rotating the scope laterally under the middle turbinate.

Third Pass

This usually requires the $30°$ (most common) or $45°$ scope. An alternative approach would be to reposition the patients head. The scope is passed along the nasal floor until the choana is reached. From here, the sphenoethmoidal recess, superior meatus and olfactory cleft can be examined.

Post-procedure Care

Once the examination is complete, one should explain both the positive and negative findings to the patients in order to help alleviate any anxiety. Future management plans should also be discussed. Both the positive and negative findings should be documented clearly in the notes with the aid of diagrams if possible. If it is possible to take photos during the examinations then these should be placed in the notes for future reference. If topical anaesthetic has been used, then the patient should be warned not to eat or drink any hot items for approximately one hour post-procedure to prevent burn injuries

5.4. Microlaryngoscopy

Setting up a manikin in the correct position for microlaryngoscopy is a clinical skill scenario which may be encountered in ST3 interviews.

It is not unreasonable for candidates to be expected to choose an appropriate laryngoscope, attach a light lead and talk an examiner through the steps of a microlaryngoscopy procedure as well as answer questions relating to indications, consent and post-operative care.

Indications

- Suspected malignancy
- Vocal fold polyps
- Vocal fold cysts
- Severe Reinke's oedema
- Laryngeal papillomatosis
- Vocal fold medialisation
- Airway surgery – arytenoidectomy, posterior cordectomy, subglottic/tracheal stenosis

Please note, surgery is rarely indicated in the management of vocal fold nodules. These lesions respond to voice therapy +/- anti-reflux therapy.

Pre-operative management and consent

Appropriate work-up for any microlaryngoscopy procedure includes an initial consultation with a speech therapist. This provides an opportunity to implement changes to the patient's voice use and for discussion of the post-operative instructions in detail.

Informed consent should include a full explanation of microlaryngoscopy and the specific indication for the patient and an explanation of the risks and complications. The latter includes: damage to teeth and soft tissues of the lips and oral cavity, bleeding, infection, temporary worsening of the airway, scarring and the need for further procedures.

Patient Position

- Patients lie supine in the 'sniffing the morning air' position.
    o The neck is flexed and the head is extended.
    o There is no requirement for the placement of a pad under the shoulders.
    o The head rests on a head ring
- A mouth guard is placed over the upper dentition, in edentulous patients this is substituted with a damp gauze swab.
- The laryngoscope is assembled and lubricated with aqueous jelly.
- The left hand is used to gently retract the lips and open the oral cavity. The laryngoscope is held in the right

hand and gently advanced through the oral cavity to the larynx.

- If the view of the anterior larynx is poor, there are several means of improving it.
    - Flexing the head of the table
    - Changing the laryngoscope to an anterior commissure laryngoscope
    - The application of sticky tape across the anterior neck to compress the cricoid cartilage.

Laryngoscopes and suspension

The best laryngoscope for each patient is the largest one that provides a good view of the larynx. There are several manufacturers of laryngoscopes, resulting in various types. Candidates are advised to familiarise themselves with the laryngoscopes used in their local hospitals and be competent in assembling them including the attachment of the light cable.

Once the appropriate laryngoscope has been chosen, the light cable is attached securely. The laryngoscope is now ready for use. Once an acceptable view of the larynx is achieved, the laryngoscope can be placed in suspension. There are several suspension systems available. The key factor when applying suspension is to tighten the suspension arm after the desired view has been seen, it must not be used to improve the view as this increases the risk of using the teeth as a lever with resultant tooth subluxation, fracture or avulsion.

In the interview setting, the manikin's teeth are likely to emit an audible click if they are used as a fulcrum to lever the laryngoscope; this must be avoided!

Figure 5.2 A ST3 Candidate preparing to perform laryngoscopy in a manikin on ENTTZAR interview course 2011

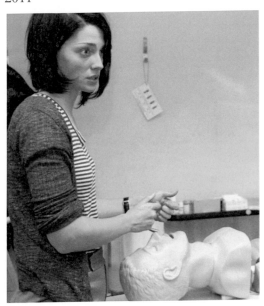

Post-operative Voice Care

There is currently no widespread consensus on post-operative voice advice. The literature reports a variation in practice, however the most commonly used regime after instrumentation is absolute voice rest for seven days. The voice is only used in emergencies, e.g. calling for help, shouting 'fire'. Patients must be advised that whispering inflicts more damage on the larynx than a normal speaking voice and is not permitted in the post-operative period.

5.5 Sutures and suturing

It is not unreasonable for a clinical skills station on sutures and suturing to appear in ST3 interview. The requirement for wound support varies in different tissues. Each tissue's healing rate determines the type of suture required.

Types of Sutures

Sutures can be classified into two types, absorbable and non-absorbable. These can be further divided into monofilament and multifilament sutures. Monofilament sutures have a single strand and tie down easily during knot formation and are less likely to harbour micro-organisms. Multifilament sutures are twisted or braided, this improves the suture's handling and tying properties, however there is an increased risk of infection including stitch abscesses.

Absorbable sutures undergo degradation resulting in loss of tensile strength as the tissues regain their original strength to keep the wound edges opposed. Natural absorbable sutures are digested by tissue enzymes, while synthetic absorbable sutures are hydrolysed in tissue fluids. Non-absorbable sutures remain at the site of placement and are walled off by fibroblasts.

Table 5.3 Absorbable sutures

Suture	Type	Tensile Strength Retention	Absorption rate	ENT Application
Polyglactin 910 *Vicryl*	Braided	75% remaining at 2 weeks 50% remaining at 3 weeks	Complete at 56-70 days	Subcutaneous closure Tying blood vessels
Polyglactin 910 *Vicryl rapide*	Braided	50% remaining at 5 days	Complete at 42 days	Subcutaneous closure
Poliglecaprone 25 *Monocryl*	Monofilament	50-60% remaining at 1 week 20-30% remaining at 2 weeks	Complete at 90-120 days	Subcuticular sutures
Polydioxanone *PDS II*	Monofilament	70% remaining at 2 weeks	Absorbed in 180-210 days	Subcuticular closure

		50% at 4 weeks 25% at 6 weeks		
Glycolide/ Lactide co-polymer *Polysorb*	Braided	80% remaining at 2 weeks 30% remaining at 3 weeks	Absorbed in 56-70 days	An alternative to vicryl
Polyester *Biosyn*	Monofilament	75% remaining at 2 weeks 40% remaining at 3 weeks	Absorbed in 90-110 days	An alternative to vicryl

Table 5.4 Non-absorbable sutures

SUTURES	TYPE	TENSILE STRENGTH	ENT Application
Surgical Silk *Silk*	Braided	Non-dissolvable because of the presence of amyloid.	Securing neck drains Securing trachesotomy tube flanges to the skin. May be used as ties.
Nylon *Ethilon*	Monofilament	No degradation	Skin closure
Polpropylene *Prolene*	Monofilament	No degradation	Skin closure
Polyester fibre (uncoated) *Mersilene*	Braided	No significant change over time	Pinnaplasty; cartilage suturing
Polyester (silicone-coated) *TI-CRON*	Braided	No degradation	Pinnaplasty; cartilage suturing

Polyester *Novafil*	Monofilament	No degradation	Skin closure

Suturing Technique

Candidates must be well versed in suturing using either an instrument or hands (Figure 5.4). The instrument tie and the two-hand tie are the most common techniques used in ENT. The detailed steps of both of these techniques lie beyond the cope of this book, but a good Basic Surgical Skill manual/course will be a useful refresher.

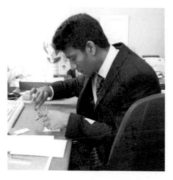

Figure 5.4 A ST3 candidate practicing suturing 2011

Suturing principles

- Pick up skin edges with a pair of toothed-forceps, but do not crush the tissue between the tips of the forceps.
- Hold needle holders with confidence grasping the suture needle about two-thirds of the way along its circumstance
- Avoid excessive tension on sutures

- Insert the needle at right angles to the tissue
- A rough guide to suture placement, is the distance from the edge of the wound should be equal to the thickness of the tissue and subsequent sutures should be placed at twice this distance, i.e. twice the depth of the tissue.

Knot tying principles

- Knots must be firm and not slip
- Keep knots as small as possible to minimise tissue reaction
- Avoid grasping the suture material itself with the needle holders

Forms of suturing

- Interrupted suture
  - o This is the placement of a single suture through tissue secured with a reef knot.
- Continuous suture
  - o This is the placement of a single suture, where only one end is cut after the first reef knot. The suture is then passed continuously through the tissue to close the wound, with a second reef knot placed at the distal end of the wound.
- Mattress suture (vertical, horizontal)
  - o This form of suture is very good for everting the edges of the wound.
  - o The needle is passed through the tissues on one side, then again through the same side, but either further along (horizontal) or deeper (vertical) and then the same two passes made on the opposite skin edge (Figure 5.5).
- Subcuticular sutures

- o This is a continuous running suture through the subcutaneous tissue. The ends of the suture are either buried, taped down or secured with a bead.
    - o

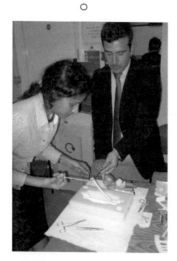

Figure 5.5 A ST3 Candidate performing mattress suture on simulated model on ENTTZAR ST3 Interview course 2011

5.6 Types of needles

Surgical needles are made from stainless surgical steel.

Round-bodied Needles

These needles are designed to separate the tissues rather than cut through them. Once the needle passes through, the tissue closes tightly around the suture needle. This provides a leak-proof suture line. A cross-sectional view of the needle is round.

ENT Application: Suturing fauces together in the management of post-tonsillectomy haemorrhage.

Cutting needles

The conventional cutting needle has a triangular cross-section with the apex of the curve on the inside of the needle. The needle is limited to cutting on its front section only. This needle will cut a pathway through tissue.

<u>*ENT Application:*</u> Skin closure

Reverse-cutting needles

This needle is also triangular in cross-section; however the apex cutting edge is on the outside of the needle curvature. There is less risk of cutting out the tissue. The reverse-cutting design of the needle results in an increased needle strength and increased resistance to bending.

<u>*ENT Application:*</u> Mucosal closure and pinnaplasty.

5.7 Tuning fork tests, audiograms & masking rules

Tuning fork test

Rinne's and Weber's tuning fork tests help us to differentiate between conductive hearing loss and sensorineural hearing loss. A conductive hearing loss may be due to any disruption of the sound transmission from the external ear to the oval window whilst a sensorineural hearing loss involves the cochlear and/or the auditory nerve. You would have learnt to perform these tests before DOHNS exam, so it is not worth describing them here. However, please remember to give clear simple instructions whilst demonstrating what you are saying. Also remember to use correct English, eg say 'which sound is louder' not 'which sound is loudest'

Weber's test

A Weber test is used to test for conductive hearing loss (Figure 5.6). Normally the tone is heard in the midline or equally on both sides. In unilateral conductive hearing loss the tone is louder in the affected ear. In a unilateral SHNL the tone will be heard louder in the better ear (i.e. the contralateral ear without the SNHL).

Figure 5.6 Demonstrating Weber's tuning fork test.

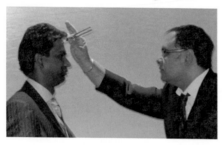

Rinne's test

The Rinnie's test compares air conduction with bone conduction (Figure 5.7). By convention a **positive** Rinne's test is normal, i.e., the tone in air conduction is louder than that in bone conduction. A positive Rinne's test may occur in patients with sensorineural hearing losses such as elderly patients with presbyacusis. Generally, patients with a conductive hearing loss will perceive the tone being louder in bone conduction compared to air conduction. Table 5.5 summarises the interpretation of the two tuning fork tests.

Figure 5.7 Demonstrating Rinne's tuning fork test

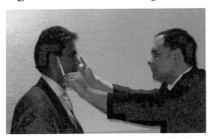

Table 5.5: Interpretation of tuning fork tests

RINNE'S	WEBER'S	INTERPRETATION
Positive bilaterally (AC>BC)	Central	Normal or bilateral SNHL (presbyacusis)
Negative on right, positive on left	Louder in right ear	CHL right ear
Negative on left, positive on right	Louder in right ear	Profound SNHL left ear ('dead' ear)
Positive bilaterally (AC>BC)	Louder right ear	SNHL left or small CHL right
Right unequivocal (AC=BC); left positive	Louder in right ear	CHL right

In an interview setting or in an examination, the actor may be prep to say that tone is the same in both air conduction and bone conduction during a Rinne's tuning fork testing. This means that there is a small conductive hearing loss present but it is not large enough to be detected by the tuning fork used. With a standard 512Hz tuning fork, it is necessary to have an air bone gap of greater than 20dB to get a positive Rinne's result. The 256Hz tuning fork is more sensitive and will result in a positive Rinne's result if the air-bone gap is greater than 15dB. A 1024Hz tuning fork is least sensitive, requiring an air-bone gap of over 30dB to produce a positive Rinne's result.

Audiograms

An audiogram is a graph with frequency (Hz) plotted on the x-axis and intensity (dBHL) on the Y-axis. However, unlike most graphs the Y-axis is plotted from the lowest intensity at the top of the graph to the highest intensity at the bottom. Frequency is listed either at the top or bottom of the graph.

Key points pertaining to Pure Tone Audiograms

I.   A pure tone audiogram (PTA) is the main behavioural hearing test for adults and children from around developmental age of four years.

II.   The thresholds of hearing for a range of tones (250Hz - 8000Hz) are deduced for each ear by the patient responding to the each tone that is heard.

III. The PTA indicates overall hearing thresholds, as well as any sensorineural or conductive elements if there is a hearing loss (Table 5.6).

IV. If noise induced hearing loss is suspected or the gap between thresholds at the higher frequencies (2-8 kHz) is greater than 20dBHL, then 3 kHz and/or 6 kHz are/is tested.

V. Bone conduction audiometry (500Hz - 4 kHz) is only required if any thresholds fall outside the normal range (-10 to +20dBHL).

VI. Any asymmetry needs investigating with masking (air-conduction or bone conduction) so that the function of each cochlea can be determined.

VII. Standardised symbols are used on a pure tone audiogram (Figure 5.7)

Table 5.6: Levels of hearing loss (rough guide)

Thresholds (dbHL)	Degree of hearing loss
0-20	Normal
21-40	mild
41-60	moderate
61-90	severe
>90	profound

Note that a dB = one tenth of a Bel (B) = 1/log intensity of sound (1B = 10dB)

Table 5.7: Symbols used in audiograms and their meanings

Description	Right ear	Left ear
Air conduction (when necessary)	◯	X
Air Conduction not masked (shadow point)	●	◤
Air conduction masked (not changed from previous test)	◕	✕
Air conduction limit, threshold not found	◯↓	✗
Bone conduction not masked	△	△
Bone conduction masked	⊏	⊐
Bone conduction limits, threshold not found	⊏↓	⊐↓
Uncomfortable loudness level	L	⌐
Uncomfortable loudness level not found	L↓	⌐↓
Sound field	~S	~S
Aided	A	A

Masking rules

Most ENT surgeons find the 3 rules of masking confusing. This is probably because of the incomprehensible text used to explain the rules. Rule 3 is the most difficult to understand because of 2 reasons (a) failure to appreciate the presence of a conductive hearing loss in the better ear and (a) failure to appreciate the effect of the presence of headphones on both ears during **air conduction** testing.

ENTTZAR team has developed a novel triangle (Figure 5.8) to explain when masking is necessary. Each side of the triangle represents one rule of masking. It is important to note the following points:

i. Masking always involves a noise given through air conduction (never through bone conduction) in the **non-test** ear.

ii. Each rule of masking applies independently at each frequency on an audiogram.

iii. When Rule 2 is invoked, the bone conduction threshold needs to be masked as opposed to rules 1 and 3 when the air conduction threshold in the *better ear* is masked.

iv. Rule 3 is only necessary when Rule 1 is not applicable, i.e. when there is a conductive hearing loss in the better ear (which is the non-test ear and therefore needs to be masked).

v. Figure 5.8 is based the air-conducted signal being delivered through a standard supra- or circum-aural earphone rather than insert earphone (inter-aural attenuation for the latter is 55dB).

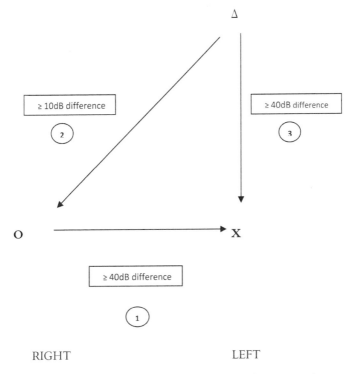

≥ 10dB difference

2

≥ 40dB difference

3

≥ 40dB difference

1

Δ

O

X

RIGHT

LEFT

Figure 5.8 A simple and effective tool that illustrates the three rules (1, 2 & 3) when masking is needed (each arrow points to the *test ear*, O unmasked air conduction right ear,

X unmasked air conduction left ear, Δ unmasked bone conduction – relevant to both ears because of the 0dB inter-aural attenuation).

5.8 Questions and Answers

Question 1. *First make a diagram of a tympanic membrane, while identifying the area you would place a grommet and ear structures one needs to be aware of during insertion. Now insert the grommet with the aid of the microscope.*

All the information in this part of the station should be given by the candidate rather than wait for prompting. A tympanic membrane sketch should indicate which ear it is from and be clearly labelled. The anatomical landmarks the candidate should point out are: the handle, umbo and lateral process of the malleus, pars flaccida, pars tensa and light reflex (Figure 5.9). The anterior and posterior malleolar ligaments could be added as well. Grommet insertion is a straightforward procedure and the classical myringotomy incision is made in the antero-inferior quadrant of the tympanic membrane. If access is difficult the grommet can be placed in the posterior-inferior quadrant. It needs to be stressed that inferior placement of grommets is safe and insertion in the superior aspect of the tympanic membrane is dangerous. Structures that one should be aware of during insertion are the auditory ossicles (should be aware of their location in the middle ear), the chorda tympani (should know its course in the middle ear and its relation to the annulus) and the promontory (as scraping its mucosa with the myringotome can lead to unnecessary bleeding). The incision should be a radial one.

Figure 5.9 Otoscopic view of a normal left tympanic membrane

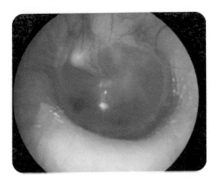

Insertion of a grommet

This part of the station examines a number of skills. Firstly it ensures the candidate is comfortable to work with the microscope and can set it up appropriately. It should be mentioned that the microscope would be initially balanced and the joints finger tight to allow for smooth co-axial movement of the surgeon with the microscope. The focal length should be checked and the inter-pupillary distance also changed according to your setting. The focus should also be checked. If for example the surgeon is wearing contact lenses, the eyepiece dial should be on zero. The light aperture should also be on the maximum (i.e. 5). Once the optimum magnification has been chosen and the microscope light is switched on, insertion of the grommet should be straightforward. You should ensure that you have scrubbed up (or are at least wearing sterile gloves). The patient should be covered and the largest size speculum inserted in the ear canal. The antero-inferior quadrant should be identified, and the incision made with the myringotomy knife. You should then ask for the grommet and crocodile forceps, mount the grommet correctly (Figure 5.10) and with a smooth movement insert it into the opening (Figure 5.11). The examiners will be looking for confidence, good communication with the scrub nurse, smooth handling of instruments, using the correct names of instruments and a professional performance overall.

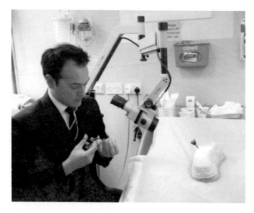

Figure 5.10 Preparing for grommet insertion on ENTTZAR ST3 Interview Course 2011

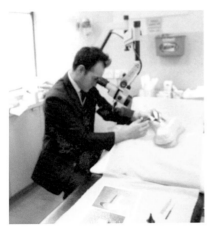

Figure 5.11 Simulation of a grommet insertion

Summary of myringotomy and grommet insertion:

- Correctly identify the ear – left/right
- Choose the correct instrument
  - Myringotomy knife, crocodile forceps, needle
- Make a myringotomy – anterior inferior quadrant, radial incision, umbo to annulus
- Identify the type of grommet
  - Shah, Shepherd, mini-grommet, t-tube
- Insert the grommet

Summary of microscope set up:

- Switch it on and increase intensity (Figure 5.2)
- Zero the eyepieces (Figure 5.3)
- Set your interpullary distance (Figure 5.4)
- Check appropriate focal length (Figure 5.5)
- Balance the microscope (Figure 5.6 a-c)

Figure 5.12 Switch it on

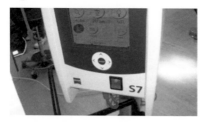

Figure 5.13 Zero the eyepieces

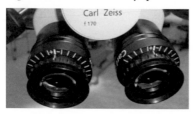

Figure 5.14 Set your interpupillary distance

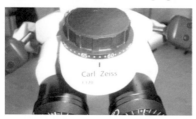

Figure 5.15 Check appropriate focal length

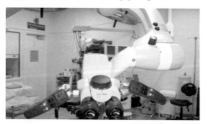

Figure 5.16 (a) Balance the microscope

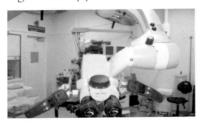

Figure 5.16 (b) Balance the microscope

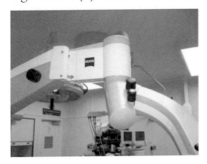

Figure 5.16 (c) Balance the microscope

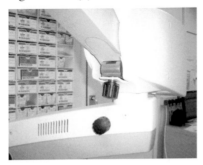

Question 2. *Perform flexible nasendoscopy and then draw a diagram of the larynx*

Flexible nasendoscopy is an essential skill for the ENT surgeon. In the exam you will have to demonstrate confidence, good handling of the instruments and good communication with the patient. The station may have an actor for the communication part of the station and a manikin for its practical aspect (Figure 5.17). At the beginning you should introduce yourself and gain verbal consent.

e.g. "Hello Mr Smith, I am Mr Argiris, one of the ENT surgeons. Would it be alright if I examined your nasal passage and voice box with this camera?"

A quick explanation of what the examination entails should also be done while preparing the cophenylcaine spray that numbs the nasal mucosa and has some vasoconstrictor effect. Before spraying the nasal airway it should be stressed that it tastes foul and that the patient should not eat and drink anything for about an hour.

e.g. "I will pass this camera into one of your nostrils. It is not painful but you find it a bit uncomfortable, that is why I have sprayed you with this local anaesthetic. If you find it uncomfortable just let me know and I will stop. I will be looking at your nasal passage, the back of your nose, throat and voice box. Throughout the procedure I will ask you to do a few things. It should all last about a minute"

Once everything has been explained and you have allowed the local to work the actual procedure should follow the sequence below. This examination is based on a patient with laryngeal pathology. Clearly if one is assessing the PNS or nasal pathology, the scope needs to be passed through both nostrils

- When holding the scope, ensure you are happy with the focus and lighting
- Put some lubricant and ask the patient to stick out their tongue in order to moist the front part of the scope
- Whichever finger you have learned to control the scope (i.e. index or thumb) just stick to that so you do not confuse yourself. Both are acceptable
- Pass the scope about 1-2cm just beyond each vestibule to identify the better nasal passage
- While inserting it ask the patient to remain calm and breath from his mouth
- Pass the scope through the floor of the nasal cavity
- Once in the PNS curve the scope inferiorly and as you advance it further down straighten it out again
- You may then ask the patient to start breathing from the nose
- Once at the tongue base, ask the patient to stick out their tongue, and then extend their chin (for better view of airway).
- Progress the scope further inferiorly, down to the larynx and ask the patient to turn his head to the right and left while looking at the piriform fossae
- Once there, obstruct patient's nose with your fingers and perform a Valsalva manoeuvre while looking at the piriform fossae.
- Inspect the rest of the larynx, including the epiglottis, aryepiglottic folds, arytenoids and vocal folds.
- Ask the patient to perform a Valsalva manoeuvre to open up the ventricles
- Ask the patient to take a deep breath in and out looking for vocal fold abduction.
- Ask the patient to say "eeeeh" looking for vocal fold adduction
- Ask the patient to count to 5 looking for vocal fold movement

- Progress scope as far down as possible to get a glimpse of the subglottis
- Remove scope and hand over to nurse for cleaning or state you would clean yourself
- You then document in the notes your findings

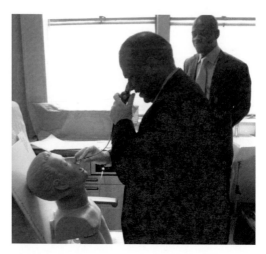

Figure 5.17 A ST 3 candidate performing FNE on a manikin at ENTTZAR ST3 Interview course 2011

Documentation

At this point you should not fall into the trap of simply drawing a larynx in a real life situation. The patient's details should be clearly written on the top. The time and date should also be recorded. The details of the medical interaction should be written legibly in the presence of the sticker indicating the use of the nasendoscope. In the case of the interview, the diagram below may be adequate (Figure 5.18).

Figure 5.18 Simple documentation of FNE findings

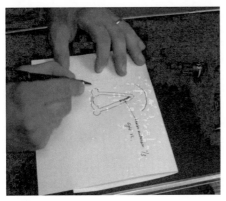

Question 3. *Describe the following audiograms (a) and (b).*

Audiogram (a)

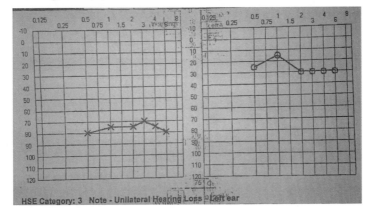

HSE Category: 3   Note - Unilateral Hearing Loss – Left ear

Answer 3 (a)

The above audiogram show severe hearing loss in the LEFT ear and mild high frequency hearing loss in the right ear. It is a bit confusing because it is not presented in the conventional way, i.e. the air conduction thresholds for left ear are plotted on the left hand side, whilst those for the right ear are plotted on the right hand side.

Audiogram 3 (b)

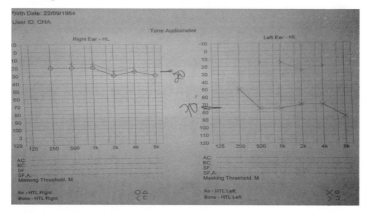

Answer 3(b)

This audiogram is actually from the same patient with audiogram 3(a) but plotted in the conventional way. It shows mild sensorineural hearing loss on the right since there is hardly any air-bone gap between air and masked bone conduction thresholds. The audiogram for the left ear shows a significant conductive hearing loss with an average air-bone gap of about 60dBHL. This is the maximum amount associated with a conductive hearing loss and likely to represent ossicular discontinuity.

Question 4. *Describe the audiograms and comment on the significance of the word recognition scores.*

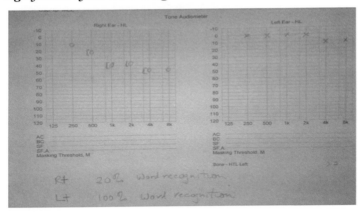

Answer 4

The audiograms show a moderate sensorineural hearing loss on the right and normal hearing on the left. Because of the poor speech discrimination on the right, the hearing loss is likely to be due to a retrocochlear lesion, such as, an acoustic neuroma.

Question 5. *Describe the audiograms. Explain the aetiology and relevant investigations needed, if the problem with his left ear occurred over night.*

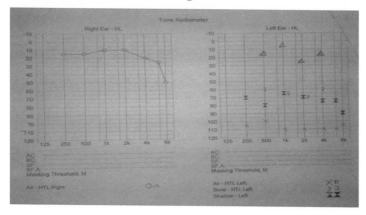

The audiograms show mild to moderate hearing loss on the right and profound sensorineural hearing loss on the left.

Aetiology: Congenital, idiopathic, trauma, infection, tumour, Menieres cholesteatoma, iatrogenic

Investigations for sudden SNHL:

MRI (CPA/IAM), FBC, U&Es, ESR, glucose, cholesterol, triglycerides, TFTs, clotting, HIV, lymes serology,

Syphilis (FTA-Abs, VDRL), ANA and RF

Question 6.   *Describe the audiogram below. What is the most likely diagnosis?*

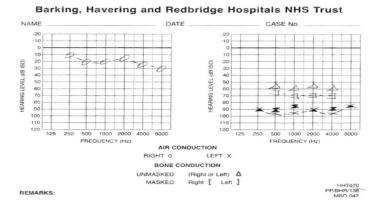

Answer 6

The audiogram of the right ear shows air conduction thresholds with average thresholds of about 20dBHL. The audiogram of the left ear shows unmasked bone conduction, masked bone conduction, unmasked air conduction and masked air conduction.

According to the Rules of Masking, the unmasked bone and air conductions should be much higher on the graph because the interaural attenuation for bone conduction is taken as zero that that for air conduction is 40 dBHL (with head-phones). For instance at 250 Hz the left unmasked bone conduction should be 10dBHL (instead of 60dBHL) because the right ear would pick up the bone conducted sound. Similarly at 250Hz the unmasked air conduction on the left side should be approximately 50dBHL (instead of 90dBHL). The joined up shaded symbols represent shadow curve★ (individual points are called shadow points). The most likely diagnosis is therefore non-organic hearing loss (NOHL).

★Shadow curve

- Is obtained when air conduction thresholds recorded for the test ear actually represent the responses of the non-test ear

- This means that a deaf ear will appear to have responses 40dBHL or more than the threshold of the non-test ear

- Masking will eliminate the shadow curve and reveal the true responses for the test ear

Question 7. *The following audiograms were taken 6weeks apart in a patient aged 35 years old. Explain what you see and what may be responsible for the hearing loss?*

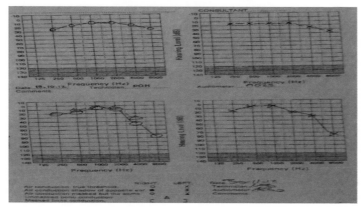

Answer 7

The audiograms at the top (taken 18/10/12) represent air conduction thresholds in the right and left ear. On the right side there is mild hearing loss at 250 Hz and 8000Hz; the thresholds at the other frequencies are within normal range (0-20dBHL). On the left there is mild hearing loss at 4000Hz and 800Hz, the thresholds at the other frequencies are normal.

The audiograms shown at the bottom (taken 30/11/12) show significant sensorineural hearing loss in the high frequencies in both ears. The most likely cause for this hearing loss in a young person is drug induced for example cisplatin or aminoglycoside antibiotics (this patient was actually on the cochleotoxic agent amikacin for resistant TB).

5.9 Additional information relevant to clinical audiology

If you are doing well it is not unreasonable to ask advanced questions or to demonstrate free field testing. The flowing information may therefore come in handy.

Free field testing

- Done by bedside
- Is a useful adjunct to PTA
- Is helpful with young children
- Fairly sensitive (good indication of HL)
- Patient can hear whisper at arms length = normal hearing (<30dBHL)
- Patient can hear conversation voice at arms length = mild to moderate HL (<60 dBHL)

- Patient can hear whisper at half of arm's length = Mild Hearing loss (between 30 and 60dBHL)

Figure 5.19 Two ways (a) and (b) of performing free field testing in adults

(a)

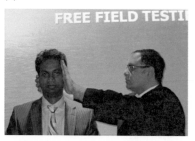

(b)

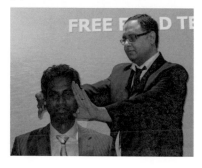

Steps for performing a PTA

I.	Otoscopy and explanation
II.	Start AC in better ear
III.	Start at 1000Hz at 60dB
IV.	Down 10dB until no response
V.	Up 5dB until response (3 out of 5)
VI.	Up and down frequencies
VII.	Repeat 1000Hz
VIII.	Same for BC

Figure 5.20 Air conduction testing

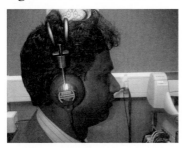

Figure 5.21 Bone conduction testing

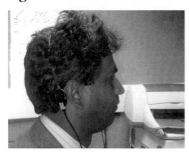

Masking dilemma

Masking dilemma occurs when the noise presented to the non-test ear crosses over to test ear and interferes with the threshold measurements. This can occur when there is bilateral large CHL (AB=60db)

Figure 5.22 Audiogram illustrating masking dilemma

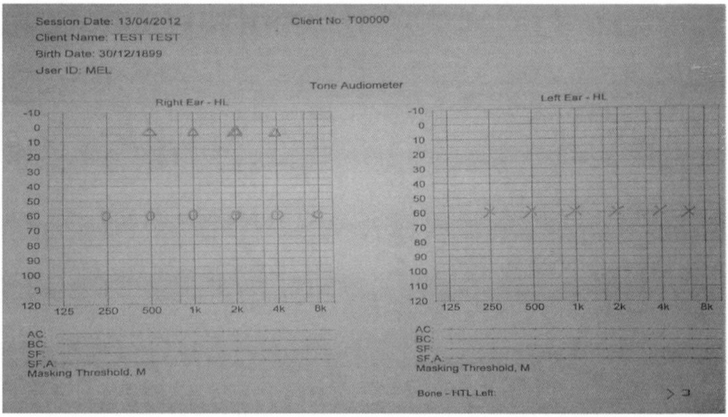

5.10 Marking Scheme

In 2012, a total of 20 marks were allocated for the clinical skill station. Clinical skills assessment involved performing and interpreting tuning fork tests (Weber's and Rinnie's) accurately, as well as interpretations of audiograms. The patient had profound unilateral SNHL. Marks were given for gelling hands, selection of tuning fork, correct use of tuning fork, giving clear concise instruction, interpretation of audiological symbols as well as for the aetiology and investigations of sensori-neural hearing as well as conductive hearing losses.

Chapter 6

Managerial Station

6.1 Overview

The management station usually involves clinical governance issues along with professional integrity and the responsibilities of a NHS employee. The modern style of interviewing has moved away from asking several short questions such as "what is the difference between audit and research?" More general and longer questions are used that aim to better test your understanding such as "what is your understanding of the term clinical governance?" If you consider most stations only last for 10-15 minutes and involve questions with long responses it is unlikely you will be asked more than three questions within the management station. In fact, as professional integrity and responsibilities of an NHS employee need to be assessed, it is unlikely you will be asked more than two questions on clinical governance. Consequently the questions you will face will either be very general so as to test that you understand clinical governance and can give examples of how you involve yourself in each of the seven pillars or will focus on the pillars that doctors are most involved in such as audit, clinical effectiveness and clinical risk management. It is still worth practising the short more traditional clinical governance questions as well though so you feel ready for anything on the day. Also be aware of the scenario based question that can cover responsibilities of an NHS employer, professional integrity and clinical governance in one question. In this chapter we will highlight the key information relevant to clinical governance, leadership and management, consent and relevant UK legislations, DVLA, Data Protection and Ethics as well as some common questions and answers.

6.2 Clinical Governance

Introduction

Clinical governance is a relatively new concept within medicine and has become common place in the medical interview. It is essential that one develops a sound understanding of clinical governance as well as examples of how it is used within the clinical workplace as the interview is usually centred on these two themes. In essence the range of potential questions that may be asked are comparatively limited, and it is hoped that once you have read this chapter and with a bit of extra work you should aim for full marks in this part of the interview.

Definition

"A framework through which NHS organisations are accountable for continually improving the quality of their services and safeguarding high standards of care by creating an environment in which excellence in clinical care will flourish" (*G Scally and L J Donaldson, 'Clinical governance and the drive for quality improvement in the new NHS in England' BMJ (4 July 1998): 61-65.*

You should be wary of reciting this definition if asked about clinical governance as it does not show understanding and in the heat of the moment certain parts of the definition might be forgotten. A much better approach would be to formulate your own answer to include the following points:

a) Clinical governance is a framework or umbrella term that encompasses a number of activities
b) It is a quality improvement process that aims to maintain and improve the quality of care delivered

c) All NHS workers are responsible for participating in clinical governance activities

d) Clinical governance provides accountability for NHS organisations.

e) It involves seven pillars – staff management, patient involvement, clinical effectiveness, information and IT, education and training, audit and clinical risk management.

Seven Pillars

The acronym SPARE IT (**S**taff management, **P**atient Involvement, **A**udit, **R**isk management, clinical **E**ffectiveness, **I**nformation, **T**raining) is commonly used to remember the seven pillars and can be a useful tool when under fire in an interview.

1. Staff management

Staff management refers to the correct recruitment and management of NHS staff, the promotion of good working standards, the retention and development of staff and ensuring underperforming staff members are managed appropriately. As doctors we are less involved with staff management but useful examples include rota co-ordinating or designing new timetables, sitting in on interviews as a junior doctor representative and being part of committees discussing issues that affect staff.

2. Patient and public involvement

Both patients and the public should be involved in important health decisions and in developing the service. Examples include the patient advice liaison service (PALS), patient surveys and patient forums. As a doctor good examples to use are patient satisfaction surveys that you collected and led to a change in practice which in turn led to improved patient satisfaction on re-survey. Other examples could be dealing with a complaint or being involved in patient outcomes.

3. Audit

Clinical audit is a quality improvement process that compares clinical practice against pre-determined criteria or standards to assess whether current practice meets levels of expected practice. It is a continuous process that follows a cycle known as the audit cycle involving six steps.

- Step 1. Identify an issue or problem
- Step 2. Identify a standard
- Step 3. Collect data on current practice
- Step 4. Compare current practice with the standard
- Step 5. Implement any changes needed to address any shortfall from the standard
- Step 6. Re-audit to ensure any changes have led to an improvement in practice

It is essential that you have a good and well thought out example of an audit that you initiated and can demonstrate that you have involved yourself in each of these steps. The final step is perhaps the most important with extra marks always allocated to those that have performed a re-audit and can demonstrate an improvement in patient care.

Why is audit important?

When answering any question that relates to importance, structure your answer into why it's important to patients, why it's important to me and why it's important to the trust.

- *Important to patients*: Improved quality of care by providing a system that highlights deficiencies, implements change and ensures the change is effective. Audit data can also be used to inform patients of standards of care that helps them make a more informed choice over which healthcare provider to attend.
- *Important to me:* The audit process improves my team working and presentation skills and helps me become directly involved in improving standards, including my own practice.
- *Important to the trust:* Audit allows the trust to be accountable and demonstrate the quality of the service or identify areas for improvement.

Problems with audit

Several key drawbacks of audit exist although when identifying a negative try and also mention a positive to balance the answer.

1. Audits are helpful in identifying a problem but less good at identifying why that problem exists although with careful data collection clues can appear as to the cause of the shortfall in standards.
2. Audits are commonly not followed up with re-audit due to turn over of staff and loss of interest once the original audit has been performed. Ways round this are to elect an audit lead from a permanent member of staff who identifies which audits are due a re-audit and highlights this to the team.
3. The results of audits and implementation of changes to practice can cause friction within a team if the outcome is not agreeable to all team members. Careful and sensitive delivery of information and good communication skills can help prevent this.

Table 6.1 The difference between audit and research

Research	Audit
Theory driven and tests a hypothesis to generate new knowledge	Practice driven that uses standards that represent existing knowledge
One off event with defined start and end points	Continuous process following the audit cycle
Always requires ethical approval	Rarely requires ethical approval
Results can be generalised and reproduced	Results are usually locally relevant
Uses a scientific patient sample	Uses a non scientific patient sample

4. Clinical Risk Management

Clinical risk management can be defined as the way NHS organisations identify, prioritise, monitor and minimise risk. When talking about clinical risk management you should try and structure your answer into activities that identify risk, activities that prioritise risk and activities that minimise risk. You should also have several examples for each of these that demonstrate your understanding and involvement.

- *Identify risk:* risk reporting – clinical incident forms, audit, complaints, whistle blowing, satisfaction survey, mortality and morbidity meetings, promoting a blame free culture.

- *Prioritise risk:* Clinical risk management office, area manager, National Patient Safety Agency, World Health Organisation.
- *Minimise risk:* Posters, protocols and checklists, pathways, training, Medicines and Healthcare Products Regulation Agency.

5. Clinical Effectiveness

Clinical effectiveness tries to ensure that all healthcare activities are designed to provide the best outcome for patients i.e. doing the right thing to the right person at the right time and getting it right the first time. Clinical effectiveness is achieved through a range of activities that all centre around the use of evidence based medicine. Activities relating to clinical effectiveness can be divided into local examples and national examples. Local examples include journal clubs and the publication and promotion of local guidelines and protocols. National examples include bodies such as NICE, National Service Frameworks (NSF) and organisations such as the Cochrane collaboration. You should prepare examples of NICE guidelines, NSF and Cochrane reviews and local guidelines relevant to your specialty and be able to talk about a journal club you recently attended.

Evidence based medicine

Evidenced based medicine (EBM) can be defined as the use of the research evidence in combination with ones own clinical judgment and expertise to guide treatment in line with the patient's wishes. Whilst EBM is not itself one of the pillars it is the underlying theme behind clinical effectiveness. A sound understanding of evidenced based medicine is therefore essential.

EBM involves several steps.

- Step 1. Determine a specific clinical question on the treatment or care of a patient
- Step 2. Search the existing literature for evidence
- Step 3. Critically appraise the evidence
- Step 4. Integrate appraised evidence into own experience and judgment incorporating the patient's wishes to guide treatment
- Step 5. Reflect on the result with the patient

It is important to understand how to appraise evidence. This is commonly achieved by using the levels of evidence that rates the strength of research evidence based on the type of study performed with level 1a providing the best evidence.

Levels of evidence

- Ia – systematic review or meta-analysis
- Ib – one or more randomised controlled trial
- IIa – well designed controlled trial without randomisation
- IIb – well designed quasi experimental study such as a cohort study
- III – Well designed non experimental descriptive study e.g. correlation study, case control study, case series
- IV – Expert opinion / case report.

One should also have a good understanding on how to appraise a randomised controlled trial. This involves several key steps.

- Step 1. Did the study ask a focused question and is it relevant to me?
- Step 2. Was the study randomised appropriately?

- Step 3. Were participants appropriately allocated to intervention and control groups?
- Step 4. Blinding – were both researches and participants blinded?
- Step 5. Were all the participants accounted for at the end of the trial?
- Step 6. Were all of the results presented?
- Step 7. Did the study have enough participants to minimise chance?
- Step 8. What statistical test was used and was the result significant.

6. Information & Information Technology

The information component of this pillar refers to the use of patient data, ensuring that it is accurate and up to date, available for audit, accessible, and kept confidential. The IT component refers to the use of information technology in improving the availability and security of patient information. Examples for a doctor to use could be using encrypted USB sticks, never taking patient information out of the hospital e.g. shredding the patient hand over sheet before leaving for home and making sure you log off from a computer terminal.

7. Education and Training

This pillar refers to the need for staff to be suitably trained for the job and to keep their skills up to date. Examples include attending courses and conferences, sitting exams, reflective practice, work-based assessments, self directed learning and appraisal. It also includes one's responsibilities as a trainer so you should not forget to include any teaching activities you have been involved in. Moreover attending teaching courses to maximise your quality of the teaching could be included as well.

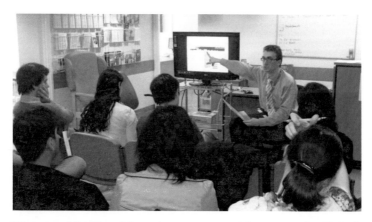

Figure 6.1 Teaching is an essential part of clinical governance (Mr Garas 2012)

General Questions

1. What is your understanding of clinical governance?
2. How do we maintain quality within the NHS?
3. If you weren't happy with the way care was delivered on your ward what would you do about it?
4. Give an example of how you prevented harm to a patient?
5. How do you ensure your treatments are effective?
6. How do you ensure standards are maintained?
7. What is your experience of audit?
8. Does research change your practice?

Short questions

1. What is the difference between audit and research?
2. Is audit important?

3. What are the disadvantages of audit?
4. How is clinical risk reported?
5. What happens to clinical incident forms once completed?
6. Who is responsible for minimising risk within your hospital?
7. In your trust who is responsible for clinical governance?
8. What is an adverse incident / near miss?
9. What is evidenced based medicine?
10. What are the different levels of evidence?
11. What are the problems with evidenced based medicine?
12. What is the difference between a standard, guideline and protocol?

Scenario based questions

1. You notice some of your consultant's decisions do not follow trust guidelines. What do you do?
2. Your colleague keeps leaving the computer without logging off and patient data open on the screen. What do you do?
3. You believe your consultant is drunk as he is scrubbing up to operate. What do you do?
4. A patient would like to make a complaint against you. How do you handle this?
5. You have lost your USB stick with important patient information on. It is not encrypted, what do you do?
6. Your colleague is not performing to a standard that you regard as acceptable. What do you do?

6.3 Leadership and Management

Management is often one of the areas most feared by trainees in the ST3 selection process. This is because of the limited experience that trainees believe they have in this field. However, there are plenty of examples in your everyday practice that can demonstrate management and leadership skills.

Firstly, it is important to identify the difference between leadership and management. Management is the *process of setting objectives and using the available resources to achieve those objectives*. Leadership, on the other hand is *influencing others to achieve common goals*, i.e. inspiring your team.

The importance of management skills in the National Health Service cannot be overemphasised, particularly these days where the political mood is encouraging clinicians to take management roles in their trusts. Indeed, the NHS Future Forum from June 2011 identifies that *"There should be clinical advice and leadership at all levels of the system and clinicians should be supported through leadership development"*. Perhaps one of the most important challenges that new registrars face is the sudden responsibility thrust upon them in terms of leading and managing a group of juniors.

The importance of management in the ST3 selection process is demonstrated by the person specification (which you should all be familiar with, and which forms the basis for the marking scheme). This has sections for leadership and team involvement, organisation and planning, decision-making and situation awareness. These skills can be readily proven in any management or leadership roles you may have undertaken.

So, how can you demonstrate evidence of leadership and management skills? The best way of breaking down management evidence is by dividing it into medical versus non-medical examples:

1. **Good documentation**: at a very basic level, this is an example of organisation and planning.

2. **Risk management**: This covers a wide range of examples, but includes incident forms, consent scenarios, discussion of the European Working Time Directive, WHO surgical checklist, and the National Patient Safety Agency. Make sure you are familiar with the GMC booklet 'Good Medical Practice'.

3. **Time management**: Any roles that you may have in terms of rota organisation/organising leave, etc. demonstrate organisational and communication skills.

4. **Resource management**: Using resources available to you is what being a registrar is all about. Examples include running an ENT emergency clinic, ensuring supplies are stocked for clinics, etc.

5. **Audit/research**: This is a vital part of clinical governance, and any involvement in audit and research will demonstrate the ability to set objectives and achieve them in a given time period. The development of any pathways/protocols within your Trust will make you stand out from the crowd.

6. **Courses**: Any courses in leadership and management are useful, as they demonstrate your insight into the increasing importance of management within the NHS. Most Trusts will usually offer local courses for a nominal price or may even be free, and there are also national courses for more senior management experience.

7. **Teaching**: Experience of teaching should be specific, i.e. regularity of sessions, number of students, level of students. Teaching provides an excellent example of management skills through the organisation and planning of sessions, delivery of sessions demonstrating communication skills, and flexible approach necessary due to the variable level of ability of the students.

Ensure you bring completed feedback forms for the interview.

8. **Societies**: Involvement in any positions in a society demonstrates not only organisational skills, but also an interest and commitment to your specialty.

9. **CMO/Darzi scheme**: This scheme allows clinicians to spend time out of their clinical training to better understand and experience the management side of the NHS, and should be strongly encouraged for those with an interest in this area.

10. **Non-medical**: Experience in any extra-curricular activities, e.g. team sports, particularly any leadership roles, or in charity work, demonstrate not only managerial potential, but also a well-rounded individual.

In the interview situation, management and leadership will be assessed throughout. However, even though management questions may appear in the portfolio station, a separate station involving management scenarios will most likely be encountered. These are often situations that you will have faced in your everyday clinical practice, e.g. a clinic running late, with nursing staff wanting to go home, and patients getting angry about the long wait, or a situation where patient safety may be compromised such as. a drunk colleague.

Some important leadership qualities to mention in all answers in the interview include:

- Ability to outline clear objectives and communicate these effectively to the team
- Ability to inspire and motivate the team
- Ability to make key decisions in stressful situations
- Flexibility to change those decisions when faced with a rapidly evolving situation

- Good communication skills and interactions with the team

At interview, the management station can also take the form of current political topics and it would be well worth your while to read up on current hot topics within your chosen specialty – for example, knowledge of training issues, subspecialisation, position papers, NICE guidelines, clinical governance, evidence based medicine, future of specialty, etc. So, hopefully you will now have a clear understanding of the difference between leadership and management, of why management is so important, and how to demonstrate evidence of leadership and management skills. Good luck!

6.4. Consent and relevant UK legislations

Consent is not a fixed point in time but a multistage process and dialogue between the patient and the surgeon and should not be relegated to the most junior member of the team. It should be taken by someone experienced with the procedure and in a non-haste environment, ideally well before any proposed procedure and accompanied by a validated patient information sheet. A discussion of the consequences of not performing the operation and potential alternative treatments must be included for balance to allow the patient to make a fully informed choice. There should be ample opportunity during and after the consultation for the patient to pose any questions.

The fundamental legal concept is to be open, informative and involve the patient in all decisions, often involving future events. A review of the revised GMC guidelines for adult and paediatric consent is important. Questions often involve consent by proxy, mental incapacity and Jehovah's Witness children requiring blood transfusions.

Table 6.2: Relevant UK legislation (summary)

Mental Capacity Act 2005: 5 Statutory Principles
Patients are assumed to have capacity unless it is established that they lack the capacity
Patients cannot be treated as unable to make a decision unless all practicable steps to help them do so have been taken without success.
Unwise decisions do not mean incapacity to make decisions
All decisions under the Act for a subject who lacks capacity must be done in their best interests
All decisions must be made in such a way as to be least restrictive to the patient and maximise the available their future choices.
'Gillick competence' criteria for the less than 18 years old
The patient has the maturity and intelligence to understand the nature and implications of treatment as assessed by the doctor.
The patient can consent to treatment if competent.
The patient may not be able to decline treatment if found to be incompetent.

Principles of robust consent

- Presume capacity and discuss risks, complications and benefits in an open and honest manner in a way designed to ensure patient understanding.
- Ensure potential relevant future events and alternative actions are considered.
- Provide options that would be least restrictive to the subject's future choices.
- Ensure decisions are voluntary.
- Respect the subject's decision and right to change their decision.
- A summary of the different ages and ability to give consent to or refuse treatment is presented in Table 6.3

Table 6.3 Different Ages and ability to give consent to or refuse treatment

Age	Can give consent	Can refuse treatment
>18years	Yes	Yes
16-18	Yes	No (in England) Yes (in Scotland)
<16	No – unless declared Gillick-competent	No- can be overridden by someone with parental responsibility

6.5 DVLA, Data Protection and Ethics

DVLA

As per GMC guidance, a physician has a duty of care to protect the public whilst also having a duty to protect individual confidentiality. The DVLA has a duty medical officer with whom advice may be taken and information confidentially exchanged. We recognise that a motor vehicle travelling at any speed or by its very bulk is a dangerous object that may maim or kill. If a patient is thought by their medical condition to have impaired ability to drive they must be advised to inform the DVLA. If contrary to this advice they prepare to drive or do drive and the physician is made aware of this the physician should act to ensure safety. Such situations most often arise when the patient's cognitive functions are impaired and in circumstances when the patients occupation or hobbies are severely restricted by the provisional cessation of driving. If an accident were to occur then a potentially criminal prosecution may be forthcoming and the patient to be protected from this must be very strongly discouraged from driving. A wise physician may then have to inform the DVLA themselves after taking medico-legal device from their defence organisation, informing the patient verbally and in writing of their advice and their need to discuss the situation with the DVLA doctor and further actions. Further advice may even be taken from the GMC helpline, but in the event of a complaint the doctor will have to justify their actions in front of the now 'lay' majority of GMC case reviewers (many of whom gain their primary income from sitting on such cases and are paid at a daily rate). Such DVLA and employment situations arise in cases of severe imbalance, sleep apnoea (especially in HGV drivers), after skull base surgery [where patients may need to stop driving for at least a year], craniofacial surgery and in recent onset epilepsy).

Data Protection

Caldecott principles (1997) for the use and sharing of patient identifiable information and data are: access must be medically justified; access must be necessary; the minimal required access to perform the task is advocated; those accessing must comply with the law and be aware of their responsibilities. An audit trail is advised.

Ethics

In all ethically compromising situations the underlying rule must be to protect patients from real or perceived harm. We do not want to see doctors who can be bribed, lie (in speech or writing), who commit crimes or who hide mistakes. Open honest and transparency is the current mantra and seems quite reasonable. Before the exams we advise you to go through the GMC handbooks, they provide broad guidance which should be followed but are scanty on the details. All gifts should be officially logged and if received be of a minor nature, this includes generous donations to hospital or personal research charities. Several hospitals now 'raid' patient funds at the end of each financial year and assurances of probity based solely upon institutional status or personal position should not be relied on. Patients should not be expected to gift their physicians for preferential treatment since we must treat patients equally in the NHS. Doctors' decisions must be based upon patients needs and not be influenced by financial inducements or profits. Competing and conflicts of interest are now often declared at appraisals so to protect against accusations of being covertly influenced or bribed. All matters pertaining to a patient's management must now be discussed with them to allow them to make reasoned choices, even if we disagree with the logic of the choice it must be respected if capacity is proven to be intact. The rights of autonomy and freedom to make choices and balanced decisions must be afforded to all patients with whom we must now share decision making (see Tables 6.2, 6.3). Sharing information even that of complications or untoward events is advocated as is formal contemporaneous documentation.

6.6 Questions and answers

Question 1. *You used a flexible nasendoscope on a patient that has now left and realise that it had not been cleaned before its use. What do you do?*

I appreciate that this is an incident that should be taken very seriously. Initially, I would gather all the appropriate information checking whether the nasendoscope was definitely not cleaned, by looking at the logbook and having a discussion with the sister in charge of the clinic. Assuming that the event was true I would take the responsibility of having to contact the patient that was scoped last and inform him/her of the event. This is a very sensitive issue and I would try and approach it a very calm and controlled way without trying to distress the patient. The content of the discussion would clearly outline the mistake that took place but also explain briefly the risks that it involves. More specifically, I would stress that even though it is very rare for infections to be transmitted through scopes, we would have to take all precautions and get in touch with the individual that had been examined before last. I would try however not to dwell too much on this as the patient would become alarmed by this and lead to unnecessary stress. I would try and address any questions or concerns the patient may have and ask whether he would like to come to hospital for a further discussion. Clearly the other patient would have to be traced as well in order to perform a battery of tests and ensure that no transmissible infection were present. After having taken this initiative I would need to inform the consultant in charge of this clinic of this event. Being a potentially serious incident and as an integral part of clinical governance I would also need to complete an incident form stating the details of this event. The purpose of this would not to put the blame on a fellow colleague or nurse, but to determine whether there was a generic flaw with the way scopes were cleaned or whether it was a one-off. Either way, the aim would be to ensure such an event would not happen again. From my side, if it were clear who was to blame I would offer personal support and reassurance to this person as a colleague friend and try to help them in any way I could.

Question 2. *You are alone in clinic as your consultant is on leave and it is running nearly 2 hours late. The staff need to leave on time and the patients are beginning to complain. What do you do?*

I appreciate that this situation would be very distressing for patients and staff and would need to be resolved quickly. I would need to initially determine whether the delay is my fault by simply taking too much time or because of too many patients. From my experience however most commonly it is the latter reason. Assuming that there are no acute issues of patient safety in this scenario I would then call the general manager explaining the situation. Clearly if overbooking was the reason, it would have to be addressed at another time. My initial goal would be to try and mobilise as many free team members as possible. Ideally fellow Registar's or senior SHOs. Foundation Year doctors, would unfortunately probably take more time than be of help because of their lack of experience. Finally if there were a consultant at hand willing to help that would be ideal as he/she would be most the productive within the limited time frame. Realistically however there would probably be an SHO at best. The next aim would be to prioritise the patients based on clinical need. I would scan through the notes and any cancer referrals (2 week wait) or other more urgent referrals would be seen on the day. I would ask the nurse to have these patients taken to a separate side of the clinic waiting area. I would then have to personally speak to the remaining patients and be frank about the situation and at the same time be apologetic and understanding. I would give them the option of staying on with a significant chance of not being seen or go to the front desk and get a new urgent appointment within the next 10 days. Surely some patients would be very unhappy about the situation and would complain. With these patients I would advise them to go to PALS through which they would be able to voice their concerns. After the session were completed, if it were clearly an overbooking issue, I would discuss this with my consultant but also raise the issue with the clinical director and general manager so it would be addressed promptly and hopefully not repeated again. I feel that on this occasion I would not fill in incident form as this issue could potentially be solved internally.

6.7 Marking scheme for the managerial station

A total of 20 marks are allocated for managerial station. Last year two different questions were asked: one on consent and the other on health and safety issue pertaining to needle stick injury. Marks were set aside for recognition of the particular problem, awareness of various protocols (GMC, MDU, Trust), and incident reporting forms. Once again 20 percent of the marks were for global assessment and fluency of answers.

Chapter 7

Structured Interview Station

6.1 Overview

The station may assess your understanding of any topic not covered in the previous stations. It may appear difficult to prepare for. The hardest aspect you will face in this station is perhaps trying to sell yourself effectively as this is neither encouraged at medical school, nor is it something you have received formal training in. Nonetheless, you need to keep in mind that you are in a competition and must make a conscious effort to individualise yourself in order to stand out from the crowd. Doing well in this station is an easy way to boost your score and therefore improve your chances of success. The following list contains examples of some of the topics which may appear in the structured interview station (note that this list is not exhaustive).

1. Research & Audit
2. Publications and Presentations
3. NICE and SIGN Guidelines in Otolaryngology
4. Out of Program guidance
5. Teaching – Evidence of contribution to the teaching and learning of others
6. Career aspiration
7. Suitability
8. Commitment to speciality
9. Awareness of consultants role

Reading the above, you may be able to draw many similarities to what you have read on the Person Specification form. This station is a chance to show how enthusiastic you are, and to demonstrate your passion for your specialty. You really need to verbalise what you have already stated on your application form and above all, make yourself stand out. Remember to speak clearly, take your time, and think before you speak. Always try and structure your answer. In this chapter we highlight the essentials of the topic listed above. In addition we have selected of ten important questions to discuss and also provided general advice on being a good competent surgeon.

Top tip: This is a competition, go for gold!

7.2 Research, audit and teaching

Person Specification relevant to academic/research skills is as follows (1):

Academic / Research Skills	Research Skills: • Demonstrates understanding of the basic principles of audit, clinical risk management & evidence-based practice • Has understanding of basic research principles, methodology & ethics, with potential to contribute to research	• Evidence of relevant academic & research achievements, e.g. degrees, prizes, awards, distinctions, publications, presentations, other achievements • Evidence of participation in risk management and/or clinical/laboratory research	Application form Interview / Selection centre
	Audit: • Evidence of active participation in audit Teaching: Evidence of contributing to teaching & learning of others		Application form Interview / Selection centre

Research

You will be required to be able to differentiate between audit and research. This may not necessarily be a question in the portfolio station but knowledge of this is essential to avoid talking about inappropriate examples. Research provides a way of dissociating yourself from others as it is likely to be an area of limited experience for many candidates. Finding a project can be difficult and seeking help from Consultants or other specialist trainees can help in this regard. Interesting case studies can be submitted to meetings such as the Semon Club, South West ENT Academic Meeting. These also count as a podium presentation. Idealistically a published article(s) will be required to score maximum marks. The mantra of start early is especially relevant here as getting publications takes time due to the review process instigated by journals. Obviously there is great variability in an individuals exposure to research and potential to participate. Nonetheless, there will always be ways of maximising what means you have at you disposal. Remember research comes in a variety of forms and levels of evidence. So by having at least one article or working progress at interview can be used to justify your position and demonstrates activity on your part.

Audit

Choose a project which you are able to talk about with enthusiasm try and avoid basic audits such as 'documentation in notes.'

You need to have demonstrated participation in audit throughout your training but will likely be questioned about something which you have done relevant to ENT. Again you will need to be aware of the principles of audit and must have participated in a second cycle thereby closing the loop and gaining maximum points. Furthermore, you need to try and make the audit 'work' for you. That is to have presented it at least at a departmental meeting and realistically at a regional/national meeting for full marks to be obtained. If it can be published anywhere then this is also beneficial. A peer reviewed article is stipulated however, it does not have to be 'The Lancet'! many online journals exist which can be helpful.

The advice given in this textbook is for the 'perfect' portfolio which may not be achievable in reality, but by striving for the best you can will only stand you in good stead for the process as it is all about competition.

Teaching

Teaching of others exhibits a number of skills/attributes required by potential trainees. A range of teaching methods can be used as examples but they must be formal i.e. not teaching medical students over coffee! Examples may include; arranging teaching sessions for epistaxis management for new Accident & Emergency doctors, regional teaching day, faculty member for ALS, anatomy demonstrating etc. To achieve marks at interview you should be aware of the differing ways of teaching (didactic, practical etc). Thereafter, you should have sought formal feedback from the session and made changes as a result. Also attending courses to demonstrate both commitment to teaching and awareness of the principles of learning are helpful. A number of courses exist for these purposes such as Teach the Teachers, teaching and medical communication etc. Teaching forms part of the GMC's Good Medical Practice guidelines and participation in it is almost mandatory as it forms an integral part of training.

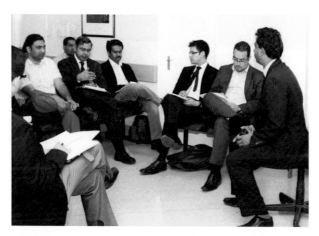

Figure 7.1 Teaching is a fundamental part of an ENT Surgeon's life

You should be able to provide clear evidence for all facets in your portfolio as well as being able to talk about them. A way of screening the quality of what you have in the portfolio is to challenge yourself to talk about it confidently.

1.http://www.yorksandhumberdeanery.nhs.uk/specialty_rec ruitment_2011/specialties/ENTST3NationalYHDLead.aspx [accessed 2/10/2011]

7.3 Publications and presentations

Publications and presentations are the Goals of the majority of the academic work that you will do in the run up to an ST3 application. They are crucial for a number of reasons.

- They allow selectors to discriminate between candidates in an objective manner.

- They give selectors a quick indication of the quality of a research or audit project – someone else will have assessed the work already and deemed it valuable.
- Involvement in a high quality audit or research project indicates various attributes ranging from the ability to write a paper, to an understanding of data protection.
- They demonstrate an area of knowledge in excess of what might be expected, which can be discussed in the answer to an interview question.
- They demonstrate enthusiasm and commitment to ENT, and show that you have the drive, resourcefulness and intelligence to bring a piece of work to completion.
- They can be used to demonstrate your involvement and understanding of a range of clinical and management issues

With respect to publications, In order to get a journal to accept a piece of work that you have submitted to them it will need to pass the process of peer review. This means that one or more experts in this field have deemed your study relevant, interesting, well designed, and clearly presented. Presentations nonetheless have to also be accepted, although usually only in abstract format. Nonetheless, you will be required to answer questions and explain your work during questions in an oral presentation, or a poster review session.

Publications and presentations can be derived from a huge number of areas. Most commonly considered is clinical activity – audits of results, reports of interesting cases, comparison between different treatments. However, publications are also derived from a wide range of issues relevant to clinical governance such as teaching programmes, patient involvement, risk management and medical staffing.

Projects leading to presentation / publication also have a range of personal involvement. They may be topics you are passionately interested in, where you think that a change in practice would be immensely beneficial to patients in your department, hospital, or throughout the country. They may also be topics which you pursue for the primary aim of submitting a piece of work for publication. Depending on the nature of your personal involvement in the piece of work, you will need to consider how this work will score on an application form, how you present this work in an interview, and how this work will affect clinical practice. Whilst marks on an application form can be quickly garnered by targeting particular work to particular journals, such work may be less beneficial when discussing your academic output in an interview. In this setting, it is more important to have completed projects in which you are intimately involved, and very aware of the intricacies of the work and its importance.

It is worthwhile to have a combination of publications, poster and oral presentations to show that you have developed the necessary skills in all of the above areas. It is important to note that although work that has been presented may then go on to be submitted for publication, the inverse is rarely true. The time that you have before application may allow or preclude using one project to score marks in a number of areas.

Desirable features in your publications:

- Is the publication in an ENT related journal, and is the journal indexed to PubMed? What is the impact factor of the journal? Journals with lower impact factors may accept publications more readily, but would be considered less prestigious.
- Original research would be preferable to a case report. It is worth considering, however, that this is a more

difficult area to give an objective score, as there are so many types of publication to consider. The relative status of reviews, meta-analysis, correspondence or case series is not clear. The application form in 2011 differentiated case reports from published research and audit. However, when discussing a piece of work in an interview question, a well-designed randomised controlled trial is the most impressive piece of work to mention.

- Are you the first author? If you are not, how many other authors are there?
- How many publications have you had accepted / published? How many of these have the above desirable features?

Desirable features in your presentations:

- What level is the presentation (local / regional / national / international)?
- What work is being presented – again, case reports will score less well.
- Are you the named presenter for the piece of work?
- Is this an oral presentation or a poster presentation? Oral presentations tend to be considered more prestigious, although this is not universal.
- Is the presentation related to ENT?
- Has the abstract of your presentation been published?
- How many presentations have you made? How many of these have the above desirable features?

Publications and presentations may be invaluable to you in the structured interview. The ability to refer to work that you have completed, and validate the quality of that work by demonstrating that it has been presented or published, allow you to demonstrate personal commitment and involvement in issues you are asked about.

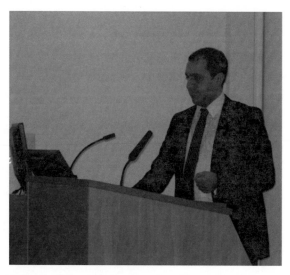

Figure 7.2 Mr Farboud explaining that presenting on a course is an important part of your professional portfolio (2011).

7.4 NICE and SIGN guidelines in Otolaryngology

There are a number of common conditions that have published guidelines within ENT that you should have used and be familiar with by the time of the interview. These are easy points to score, with questions having come up repeatedly within different stations.

NICE guidelines for surgical management of children with otitis media with effusion (Issue date February 2008)

Pathway for children with suspected OME

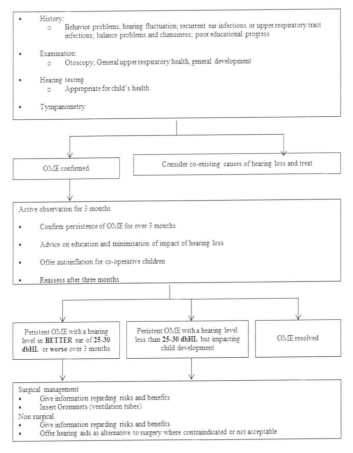

Adenoidectomy:

- Should not be performed in the absence of persistent or frequent upper respiratory tract symptoms

Other Treatments

- There is no conclusive support for the following treatments: antibiotics, antihistamines, decongestants, steroids, homeopathy, cranial osteopathy, acupuncture, dietary modification, immunostimulants, massage

Pathway for children with Down Syndrome

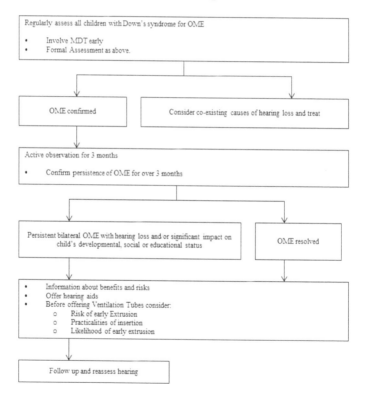

Pathway for children with Cleft palate

- The co-operation of local ENT services proficient in managing children with cleft palate with the regional multidisciplinary cleft lip and palate team is emphasized initially along with the formal assessment for OME.

- Should bilateral OME be confirmed, a waiting period of a further 3 months is recommended
- If bilateral OME persists
    o Give Information re: risks and Benefits of treatment
    o Offer Ventilation tubes as alternative to hearing aids
    o Insert ventilation tubes at the time of primary closure of cleft palate ONLY after audiological and otological assessment.

Nice Guidelines for Cochlear implantation for children and adults with severe to profound hearing loss

(Issue date: January 2009; Review date February 2011)

Cochlear implantation should only be considered for both adults and children as part of a multidisciplinary team assessment following a valid trial of an acoustic hearing aid for at least 3 months.

Criteria for unilateral cochlear implantation

- Patients with severe to profound hearing loss that do not receive adequate benefit from conventional hearing aids
    o Definition of severe hearing loss – hearing levels worse than 90dbHL at 2 and 4 kHz without acoustic hearing aids
    o Definition of adequate benefit
        ▪ Adults: score of 50% or greater in Bamford-Kowal-Bench sentence testing at a sound intensity of 70db SPL

- ▪ Children: Speech, language and listening Skills appropriate to age, developmental stage and cognitive ability

Criteria for Bilateral Cochlear implantation

- Recommended for the following patients with severe to profound hearing loss that no not receive adequate benefit from conventional hearing aids

  - o Children

  - o Adults who are blind or have other disabilities that increase their reliance on auditory stimuli as a primary sensory mechanism for special awareness

- Sequential bilateral cochlear implantation is not recommended as an option for people with severe to profound deafness

*NICE interventional procedure guidance – Suction Diathermy Adenoidectomy (*Issue date: December 2009)

- Current evidence on the safety and efficacy of suction diathermy adenoidectomy is adequate to support the use of this procedure provided that normal arrangements are in place for clinical governance, consent and audit.

- This procedure should be carried out only by surgeons with specific training in the use of diathermy for adenoidectomy because thermal damage to surrounding tissues can, rarely, cause Grisel's syndrome (subluxation of the atlantoaxial joint

Scottish Intercollegiate Guidance Network (SIGN) – Management of sore throats and indications for tonsillectomy
(Issue date: April 2010)

Guidelines for tonsillectomy

- Watchful waiting is more appropriate for children with mild sore throats
- Tonsillectomy is recommended for recurrent severe sore throat in adults
- Indications for tonsillectomy include
    - Sore throats are due to acute tonsillitis
    - Episodes of sore throat are disabling and prevent normal functioning
    - Seven or more documented and treated sore throats in the preceding year
    - Five or more such episodes in each of the previous two years
    - Three or more episodes in each of the preceding three years
- There are situations in which tonsillectomy may be appropriate outside of these criteria, ultimate judgment must be made by the appropriate healthcare professionals
- If in doubt, a six month waiting period is recommended.

Postoperative care

- Routine use of antiemetic drugs is recommended
- NSAIDS are recommended as part of postoperative analgesia to reduce PONV
- A single dose of dexamethasone is recommended to prevent post operative vomiting in children undergoing tonsillectomy or adenotonsillectomy

- A single dose of 10mg dexamethasone may be considered to prevent nausea and vomiting in adults

References

1. OME guidelines accessed via the world wide web on 10/10/2012 at 18:00 via http://www.nice.org.uk/CG60

2. Suction diathermy: accessed via the world wide web on 10/10/2012 at 18:00 via http://www.nice.org.uk/guidance/IPG328

3. Cochlear: accessed via the world wide web on 10/10/2012 at 18:00 via http://www.nice.org.uk/guidance/TA166

4. Sign guidelines: accessed via the world wide web on 10/10/2012 at 18:00 via http://www.sign.ac.uk/guidelines/fulltext/117/index.html

7.5 Out of programme guidance

Overview

Specialty Trainees may take a period Out Of Programme (OOP) to pursue research or other appropriate activities, which has been agreed formally by the Dean, whilst retaining a National Training Number (NTN). The trainees will need to discuss this with their Training Programme Director (TPD) and Educational Supervisor.

Periods out of programme may count towards the award of a Certificate of Completion of Training (CCT) - this should be discussed with the Specialty Training Committee (STC) Chair and the relevant College.

Table 7.1 Explanation of relevant acronyms

Acronyms	Explanations
OOPT	**Out Of Programme for approved clinical Training** This is time out of programme for approved clinical training in a post which already has prospective approval from the GMC but is not part of the trainee's specialty programme.
OOPE	**Out Of Programme for clinical Experience** This is time out of programme for clinical experience in a post which will not count towards the award of a CCT as it is not approved by the GMC but may benefit the doctor or support the health needs of other countries. OOPE will normally be for a period of one year, but in exceptional cases may be extended to 2 years with agreement

	from the Postgraduate Dean.
OOPR	**Out Of Programme Research**
	Time out of programme for research. OOPR will not normally exceed a period of 3 years and trainees in their final year of training will not normally be granted OOPR. GMC approval is not required if the OOPR does not count towards CCT.
OOPC	**Out Of Programme for Career break**
	Time out of programme for a planned career break. OOPC is normally limited to a period of 2 years but may extend in exceptional cases with agreement from the Postgraduate Dean. It may be taken after starting a training programme but not normally until at least one year has been completed.

It is important for prospective applicants to take in to account the following principles before making an application for time OOP.

1. Trainees requesting OOP must apply to the Deanery at least 6 months prior to the projected start date. Trainees should also contact the HR and Pensions Departments at their Trust when considering time OOP as it is important to make sure OOP will not affect maintaining their license.

2. Trainees will not normally be allowed to take time OOP in the final year of training other than in exceptional circumstances.

3. For OOPT / OOPR requests (may count towards CCT where prospective GMC approval obtained) For OOPT

/ OOPR applications, once the above documentation has been received and reviewed an application will be made by the respective Deanery for prospective GMC approval where the Head of School/Specialty Associate Dean is willing to endorse the application. Approval will be granted only once GMC approval has been received.

4. A maximum of 3 years out of clinical training will be allowed. Extensions to this will only be allowed in exceptional circumstances.

5. Six months notice must be given to the STC Chair / Training Programme Director of any changes to the anticipated date of return to the programme. Failure to do this may result in delayed re-entry to the programme or being allocated to another programme.

6. The respective Deanery must be given an up-to-date contact address and e-mail address throughout the duration of the OOP placement.

References

1. Out of programme guidance. Sections 6.66 to 6.88 of the 'Gold Guide' June 2010. This can be downloaded from the MMC website

   http://www.londondeanery.ac.uk/specialty-schools/specialties-contractual/the-gold-guide

2. http://surgicalcareers.rcseng.ac.uk/trainees/st3-and-beyond/oope

3. http://www.jcst.org/mmc_trainee_info/mmc_trainee_inf o/takingtimeout_html

7.6 Commitment to specialty

This is your opportunity to stand out, show your qualities and drive to go the extra mile for your career. At the bare minimum, the person specification expects you to demonstrate the following in relation to your commitment to ENT:

Commitment To Specialty	Learning & Development:	Extracurricular activities:	
	• Shows realistic insight into otolaryngology and the personal demands of a commitment to surgery • Demonstrates knowledge of the surgical training programme & commitment to own development • Shows critical & enquiring approach to knowledge acquisition, commitment to self-directed learning and a reflective/analytical approach to practice	• Achievements relevant to otolaryngology, including elective or other experience • Attendance at, or participation in, national and international meetings relevant to otolaryngology	Application form Interview / Selection centre References Interview / Selection centre

You will have already demonstrated evidence of prizes, courses, teaching and presentations within the relevant sections. Try including some of the following:

- Relevant Elective Experience
- Visits to other centres of excellence / ENT Taster Weeks
- ENT Charity work/travel
- ENT Bursaries/Prizes
- Memberships of relevant ENT bodies/Committees

Elective Experience

If you have performed an ENT/surgery specific elective this is an excellent opportunity to demonstrate commitment to your specialty at an early stage. Within your portfolio, you could include photos of procedures seen, a log book, evidence of a bursary, publications and written feedback from key supervisors.

ENT Charity work

This is something that is more difficult to arrange at short notice. However, if you are reading this advance of your application, look into attending a surgical charity trip abroad, such as cleft palate work or ear camps.

Within the portfolio you could include a log-book, photos, evidence of bursaries and relevant publications.

Taster Weeks/Visit to Centres of Excellence

This does not require travel abroad. There are plenty of centres of excellence within the UK, where you can arrange a taster week. Ensure you gain written feedback as proof of attendance to include in your portfolio

Bursaries and Prizes

Any relevant ENT specific travel bursaries or prizes should be included here. These can include medical school prizes or elective bursaries. Useful websites to find out about bursaries include the Royal College of Surgeons, Royal Society of Medicine (RSM), and Association of Otolaryngologists in training (AOT) websites. Examples include: Educational bursaries (RCS); Ian Mckay Essay prize (RSM); Poster prizes at conferences (BACO/CAPAG); presentation prizes at conferences (ASIT, Semon Club)

Membership of ENT Committees or Societies

Becoming a member of relevant societies facilitates attendance at key academic and social events, networking with seniors and peers, gleaming of key information in informal settings; whilst demonstrating commitment to ENT.

The 'Association of Otolaryngologists in Training' (AOT) is especially worth joining. Try to attend their annual conference, where vital tips can be obtained on training and the future of ENT.

Become a committee member if you are that way inclined. This is a great way to develop your skills in team-work, communication, organisation & planning and management. For example, becoming a member of the RSM medical student committee. Ensure any feedback and evidence is included within your portfolio.

The RSM Otorhinolaryngology section holds monthly Friday meetings, which are fantastic learning and networking opportunities. Try to book study leave well in advance so you can attend some of these meetings. Other associations or committees you may wish to consider joining are ENT UK, the British Medical Association, Women in Surgical Training, your hospital mess committee, core surgery deanery as a trainee representative, BAMMBino (British Association of Medical Managers).

Non-ENT Extra-Curricular Activities

One candidate in 2011 was asked: 'Why haven't you got any extra curricular activities in your portfolio?' It is thus important to highlight your work-life balance, extra-curricular skills and unique interests.

Music and Sport

Music and sport demonstrate skills in teamwork, leadership, communication, organisation/planning, hand eye co-ordination and commitment. Ensure you demonstrate evidence of your sporting achievements be it international, national or local.

For example raising money for charity through sporting activity, organising university ski trips, and musical interests. Such as playing instruments in an orchestra or band are all positive activities. Other areas you may wish to include are language skills, IT skills, other charity work and travel.

In summary, be pro-active and focused in everything you do in your career; utilising your time well. Ensure you keep evidence for everything, gaining written feedback where possible. Try to think outside the box, which will make your portfolio easy, enjoyable and interesting to read for the examiners.

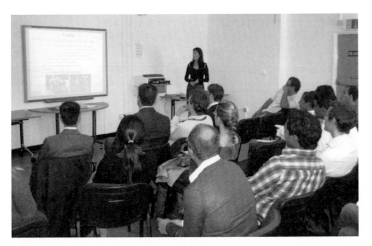

Figure 7.3 Anna Slovick explaining to ST3 candidates the importance of travelling as part of extra-curricular activities (2011).

Top Tips: - **Useful websites:**

BRINOS – See www.brinos.org.uk

AOT- http://www.aotent.com/awards.html

RSM- http://www.rsm.ac.uk/academ/awards/index.php

ENT UK- http://www.entuk.org/

7.7 Questions and answers

Question 1. *Tell me about clinical governance?*

In addition to comments regarding clinical governance in general, the answer to this question may include a comment such as '… I have demonstrated my commitment to the principles of clinical effectiveness, audit and teaching by auditing our management of epistaxis and instituting an education programme to develop the clinical skills of new A&E SHOs at our hospital. A repeat cycle of audit has demonstrated that this has improved our hospitals' management of this common and important condition. These findings were presented and discussed at a national ENT meeting in order to disseminate the findings should clinicians in other hospitals wish to address this area.' Here, additional marks are achieved by referring to your own experience in a number of areas of clinical governance, and then validating the quality of this work by showing that it has been presented nationally

Question 2. *Tell me about your involvement in management*

Part of your answer may include a comment such as "….Furthermore, in collaboration with ENT departments throughout the country, I have undertaken a study of the contributory factors in patients not attending outpatients departments. This has been published in An ENT Journal, and by changing our booking system, has allowed us to arrange follow up more effectively." Not only has have you demonstrated a role in management, you have also demonstrated that you have effected change to the benefit of the department.

Question 3. *How have you been involved in teaching?*

Practical experience of teaching medical students and other clinicians will clearly form the main part of an answer, however the answer can be improved by a brief comment such as "I have conducted a survey of medical students opinions of ENT teaching, and have highlighted that many feel that after their attachment they still have limited experience in performing ENT examinations. I presented this finding locally in order to emphasise to the department the importance of practical experience for our students." This demonstrates that you collect feedback, assess your students' educational needs, and are responsive to teaching requirements. Furthermore, by demonstrating both practical experience of teaching and the capacity to organise and design treatment in evidence based fashion, a more detailed knowledge of all that is required to teach is demonstrated.

Question 4. *What is the pathway from ST3 to Consultant?*

The way to start your answer is to make a bold statement.

"Higher Surgical training spans from ST3- ST8 and the training to become a consultant is a competency based scheme"

Then elaborate. You need to get relevant buzzwords in to score highly.

The objective of training is to finish as a highly skilled, competent, emergency safe surgeon and with a Certificate of Completion of Training (CCT) symbolising that you are the finished product. This represents the end point of training and is usually achieved once all competencies have been achieved.

You need to illustrate this answer by talking about *competency*. It is important to stress this word as all the Work Based Assessments (WBAs) test this. These include Case Based Discussions (CBDs), Clinical Examinations (CEX), Direct Observed Procedures (DOPs), Procedure Based Assessments (PBAs) and Multi Sourced Feedback also known as the Peer Assessment Tool (PAT) or 360 degree assessment. You need to know what each one assesses, how they work and how many you need. In Higher training, you need to be doing approximately 40 assessments a year, including one PAT. This equates to about one a week. Approximately half to a third should be done with a Consultant.

Type of assessment	Description
Case Based Discussion (CBD)	The method is particularly designed to test higher order thinking and synthesis as it allows assessors to explore deeper understanding of how trainees compile, prioritise and apply knowledge
	In-depth discussion between the trainee and assigned educational supervisor about how a clinical case was managed by the trainee; talking through what occurred, considerations and reasons for actions.
	By using clinical cases that offer a challenge to the trainee, rather than routine cases, the trainee is able to explain the complexities involved and the reasoning behind choices they made.
Clinical Evaluation Exercise (CEX)	The CEX is a method of assessing skills essential to the provision of good clinical care and to facilitate feedback.
	It assesses the trainees' clinical and professional skills on the ward, on ward rounds, in Accident and Emergency, or in outpatient clinics.

Procedure Based Assessments (PBAs)	PBAs assess trainees' technical, operative and professional skills in a range of specialty procedures or parts of procedures during routine surgical practice up to the level of CCT. PBAs provide a framework to assess practice and facilitate feedback in order to direct learning
Direct Observation of Procedural Skills in Surgery	DOPS are used to assess the trainees' technical, operative and professional skills in a range of basic diagnostic and interventional procedures, or parts of procedures, during routine surgical practice and facilitate developmental feedback. DOPS is used in simpler environments and procedures and can take place in wards or outpatient clinics as well as in the operating theatre

You need to mention the role of the Deanery, the Special Advisory Committee (SAC), Royal college of Surgeons (RCOS) and ISCP and how they interplay in laying out the Curriculum and implementing and supporting the training.

Acronym	Organisation
JCST SAC	The Joint Committee on Surgical Training Specialist Advisory Committee (in Otolaryngology). They decide the curriculum and training goals for each year of higher surgical training
RCSE	The Royal College of Surgeons of England • Supervises training of surgeons in approved posts • Provides educational and practical workshops for surgeons and other medical professionals at all stages of their careers • Examines trainees to ensure the highest professional standards (FRCS)
The ISCP	The Intercollegiate surgical Curriculum Project and it houses the agreed curriculum from the SAC and JCST and acts as a platform for interaction between trainees and trainers.
NHS Deanery	Each is a regional organisation responsible for postgraduate medical and dental training. As of June 2008 deaneries are regarded under UK law as employment agencies, and so are subject to the appropriate UK law

Progression depends on passing an annual review or Annual Review of Competence Progression (ARCP) previously known as the Record of In training Assessment (RITA). This means having completed the required assessments, doing research, publications, teaching, audit, basically demonstrating reaching the goals laid out in your learning agreement, and showing competence continuing improvement and progression in line with the curriculum.

ARCP Outcomes (ISCP 2008)

1. Trainee is achieving progress and competencies at the expected rate
2. Development of specific competencies required – additional training time not required
3. Inadequate progress by the trainee – additional training time required
4. Released from training programme with our without specified competencies
5. Incomplete evidence presented – additional training time may be required

Gained all required competencies; will be recommended as having completed the training programme and for an award of a CCT or CESR

(From www.iscp.ac.uk)

If you are not on the ISCP, then enrole, and find out more about it. It is not mandatory to be a member for the ST3 interview, but all your competitors will be, so I would get involved early. It will give you a better insight in to what it's all about. It is a requirement for Core trainees, and is mandatory for Higher Training. Enrolling on it demonstrates commitment to specialty. It is the platform for learning and provides the interface between you and your assessors and supervisors to record your assessments, learning agreement, Personal Development Plan (PDP), log your teaching activity, publications, audit, and there is even a reflective learning section so you can document encounters that you have learned from and feel like you want to reflect on.

Surgical logbook

Trainees are expected to log all operations undertaken and to produce this at the ARCP. There is quite specific numbers of procedures that need to be completed in the logbook to be eligible for CCT. Although this information is not essential to know, being informed will look good at the interview. Elogbook.org is now the preferred way to log surgical procedures. It highlights strengths and weaknesses. Each procedure details at what level of involvement you had, there is a chance to log the operation notes and any relevant complications for reflective practice.

JCST Recommendations (2010)

- at least 10 Mastoid Operations as only scrubbed surgeon

- 10 major neck operations as main scrubbed surgeon

- 10 tracheostomies

- 10 Paediatric Endoscopies as main surgeon

- 10 Septorhinoplasties

- 10 FESS as only scrubbed surgeon

- 10 removals of Foreign Bodies from airway.

It must provide confirmation that you have undertaken 2000 operations during the six years of training and all areas of specialist interest must be demonstrated by advanced surgical or medical experience in logbook

Question 5. *How may you enhance your training and experience prior to taking a consultant post?*

If you get this question it's a second chance to try and explain the positive indicators. In this interview station the candidates may struggle to express the information the interviewers want. Have a framework or structured answer to fall back on. Try and think outside the box, its not all clinic and theatre. Out-of program activity is varied and exciting, try and convey your enthusiasm by personalising your answers.

If you get asked this kind of question, it is a lifeline to talk more on the subject to try and score more points. It is another opportunity to talk about things involved in training that will make you stand out as a candidate and make you attractive to employers at the end of training.

You need to be aware of fellowships and research opportunities as out of program activities in the last few years before CCT. Personalise your knowledge by describing any fellowship that you have heard of and that you want to go on, or you could mention any research aspirations that you have such as an MD or Post Grad diploma in Medical Education (PgMedEd).

Fellowships can be undertaken pre and post CCT, and can be within a deanery, outside your deanery, or internationally.

Research PhD MD

Some candidates may be very keen to get involved with research. This is another out of program activity and is very involved. Expect to take at least 2 years for an MD, a year for an M.Phil or M.Sc and up to 3 – 4 years including writing up for a PhD. It is not something that should be undertaken lightly as it involves commitment, patience and dedication.

Reflective practice

For extra points you can talk about this subject. This is a hot topic at interview and a knowing about it demonstrates insight in to how you can enhance your training in the light of reduced hours due to the European Working Time Directive.

- ♦ Reflective thinking: the process of creating and clarifying the meaning of experience (past or present) in terms of self (self in relation to self and self in relation to the world.)" [2]
- ♦ Reflective thinking is a part of the critical thinking process referring specifically to the processes of analyzing, evaluating, and making judgments about what has happened.[2]
- ♦ Reflective writing: Reflective writing is writing which involves '… consideration of the larger context, the meaning, and the implications of an experience or action' [3]
    - ♦ In medicine you are required to produce reflective writing in order to learn from educational and practical experiences, and to develop the habit of critical reflection as a future health professional.

Reflective writing may be based on:

- • description and analysis of a learning experience
- • description and analysis of a past experience
- • review of your learning or course to that point
- • description and analysis of a critical incident.

Table 7.2 Positive and negative indicators

Positive indicators	Negative indicators
• knows the structure and mechanism for progression on the ENT training scheme	• Is unaware of structure of ENT training
• identifies that it is a competency based scheme	• Unable to identify the role of ISCP
• knows the role of the ISCP website in training	• Doesn't describe competency based training
• Identifies the possibilities of research and fellowship training	• Unaware of research or fellowships to enhance training expectation

In the structured interview, there are specific positive and negative indicators the interviewers have before them that guide them when they are asking their questions, these should be borne in mind.

Question 6. *What teaching skills do you have?*

This is another time to show how you have developed skills in teaching. You can divide this in to formal and informal training. Some candidates will have done a Post Graduate Diploma in Medical Education or a Royal College of Surgeons *Train the Trainers* Course. There are other more informal examples of teaching experience like mentoring,

Medical Student bedside teaching, and anything that involves teaching outside of medicine (e.g. swimming instructor). What is relevant here is to structure your answer carefully and personalise your answer. If you have organised a regional training day or departmental teaching it is important to convey all this information. The aim is to demonstrate that you have skills and that the skills are varied and adaptable. It is not important that you have every course available on your CV, but formal teacher training is a definite bonus, and may give you the edge over the opposition. Informal teaching skills show aptitude and that you have experience and ability.

Question 7. *Give an example of a particularly excellent teaching session that you have been part of as either a teacher or a pupil and explain why it was so good?*

This is a chance to really shine. It is an opportunity to demonstrate that you know something about the cycle of learning and that you can demonstrate that you have a teaching style that can be tailored towards your target audience. If you can mention the Kolbs learning cycle and that you tailor your teaching to anticipate the target audiences learning needs with respect to the Kolbs cycle, you will not only demonstrate understanding, but also you will impress the examiners. Pick a good teaching experience that demonstrates you understand the learning cycle. It may be a lecture that was followed by a workshop that was then followed by an actual surgical experience, that you reflected on and was a positive experience overall. Whatever you choose, either as a teacher or a pupil, be sure to individualise your answer, be enthusiastic and try and sound positive.

Kolbs Learning Cycle [4]

Figure 7.4 The Kolbs learning cycle

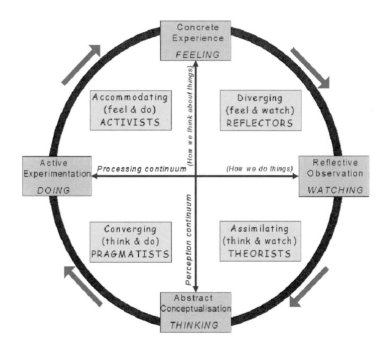

Table 7.3 Positive and negative indicators

Positive indicators	Negative indicators
• Able to identify teaching skills such as communication, explanation and demonstration • Aware of the need for preparation, clarity,	• Unaware of different qualities required for teaching successfully • Has no awareness of how to prepare a

identification of learning objectives, summarising, reflection and review at the end of any teaching session
- Aware of the importance of feedback
- Able to identify excellent teaching experience
- Able to explain what was excellent about teaching described above

teaching session or to deliver teaching
- No awareness of importance of feedback
- Unable to identify an excellent teaching situation
- Unable to demonstrate what was excellent about above teaching training experience

Question 8. *What standards of practice do you aspire to?*

This is a chance to talk about Evidence Based Medicine (EBM) and guidelines that you know about and adhere to. They may probe you and ask you the difference between a guideline, a standard and a protocol. They are defined below. At this point you could personalise your answer by talking about a specific guideline that you know about and that you adhere to, for example NICE guidelines on the management of Otitis media with Effusion. Be prepared to quote guidelines that are relevant to your day to day practice and be able to point out weaknesses and areas where you think they could be improved.

A **medical guideline** (also called a clinical guideline, clinical protocol or clinical practice guideline) [5]

A document with the aim of guiding decisions and criteria regarding diagnosis, management, and treatment in specific areas of healthcare.

Modern medical guidelines

	are based on an examination of current evidence within the paradigm of evidence-based medicine. They usually include summarized consensus statements on best practice in healthcare.
Standard of care:[6]	**1.** A diagnostic and treatment process that a clinician should follow for a certain type of patient, illness, or clinical circumstance. Adjuvant chemotherapy for lung cancer is "a new standard of care, but not necessarily the only standard of care." (New England Journal of Medicine, 2004) **2.** In legal terms, the level at which the average, prudent provider in a given community would practice. It is how similarly qualified practitioners would have managed the patient's care under the same or similar circumstances. The medical malpractice plaintiff must establish the appropriate standard of care and demonstrate that the standard of care has been breached.
Protocol [7]	A set of rules followed by providers such as doctors and

nurses. Often considered to be stricter than a guideline, and to carry more weight with the law. A protocol is a fixed list of rules that are followed without deviation for example in order to treat a hospital acquired pneumonia, a microbiology department protocol would be followed.

Question 9. *What is the role of a Consultant?*

It is sometimes forgotten when applying for ST3 posts that the ultimate goal is a Consultant's post. The purpose of the recruitment process is to find candidates who are trainable, emergency safe and highly competent. This may sound obvious, but in a subspecialty oriented field like ENT, this objective should be considered carefully. In light of the current job market for CCT holders, interviewers will be looking for potential candidates who are an all-rounder in terms of their ability and skill, and also their potential to fit in to departments depending on the clinical need.

This question can be answered in a few ways. The role can be divided in to Clinical and Non Clinical duties.

The clinical role can include

- Running dedicated theatre lists
- Clinic sessions
- In-patient care
- Team working especially MDT attendance and contribution (head and neck, thyroid, skull base)
- Triaging referrals

- Subspecialist activity (e.g. facial plastics, neurotology, anterior skull base, joint clinics, joint theatre with other specialties)

Non-clinical roles include

- Managerial tasks, chairing meetings, Departmental Clinical Lead
- Developing and maintaining services, Head and Neck cancer services
- Education and training
- Research supervisor
- Acting as a mentor, medical students, SPR's, SHO's
- CPD- audit, attending conferences, Risk assessment

If you look at the job plan for most consultants it is divided into Programmed activities (PA) and Supported Programmed activities (SPA).

Consultants have a clinical obligation to attend clinics and attend and run theatre lists. This equates to approximately 7 sessions per week, the equivalent of 7.5 PAs in managerial speak.

SPA duties varies from person to person depending on the job plan but may include many of the domains covered by clinical governance namely

- Teaching –from nurses to medical students and even Consultant colleagues and GP's
- Clinical supervision
- Writing reports/references
- Attending committee meetings/trust board meetings
- Business planning
- Advising and communicating with senior managers

It is worth noting that although as clinicians we are always learning, and have to prove this with annual reviews and soon Revalidation, when you become a Consultant you are no longer a trainee. Therefore you assume a position of responsibility that oversees many others. The decisions that you make or that are made in your name mean that you are ultimately responsible and accountable for your actions. This has implications in civil law, and needs be borne in mind.

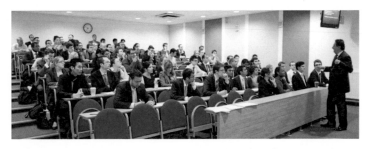

Figure 7.5 Lecturing is an essential role of a Consultant (Prof Narula at ENT ST3 interview skill course 2012).

Table 7.4 Positive and negative indicators

Positive indicators	Negative indicators
• Candidate understands all clinical aspects of a consultant ENT surgeon job plan • Is aware of non clinical roles undertaken by a consultant ENT Surgeon • Able to describe areas of subspecialisation within ENT • Identifies importance of team based working including Multi Disciplinary Team working	• Unable to describe clinical aspects of a consultant ENT surgeon job plan • Unaware of any other roles a consultant ENT surgeon undertakes • Unaware of areas of subspecialisation within ENT • Fails to mention any aspect of team working

Question 10. *Is there a role for the generalist in ENT?*

This is a difficult question to answer and in light of what has already been mentioned, the general consensus currently is to adopt a fairly neutral, balanced position. The training for registrars and the new curriculum is supposed to be general in content. Trainees are supposed to be emergency safe and highly competent in all areas of ENT at the end of the SPR years. The idea is that a new consultant should be versatile enough through their training to fit in to a department, allying their own skills to the demands of the role. For a District General Hospital, the needs may be more towards a generalist, however in a University teaching hospital; there may be more of a research, teaching, and subspecialty requirement. When answering this question it is important to present a balanced argument and to use examples. In continental Europe, Doctors are only trained to a level where they can manage emergencies, and routine operations. This is sufficient for them to begin their own practices. Should they desire further training then this can only be achieved as Fellows in University teaching hospitals, with specific mentorship. The current feeling in ENT is that trainees should avoid subspecialisation early on as they need a balanced broad based experience in surgical ENT.

When answering this question the candidate should avoid wishing to be a generalist, as this may come across as having a lack of ambition.

From a Government workforce planning point of view, they are looking to create a cohort of junior consultants that are fit for purpose and suitable for generalist type work. At the start of your career it would be acceptable to declare that you wanted to be a generalist in ENT with a sub specialist interest in Otology/Rhinology/Paediatrics although beware of coming across as too one dimensional.

7.8 Concluding remarks

In order to succeed in the national selection process, you need to start believing in yourself and know that what you are about to do is absolutely achievable. The way to do this is to start to intellectualise the situation. Once you can visualise your goal, and you have your basic attitude to the situation in-check, then you can start to really make some headway and prepare.

In 2000 the competition ratio for entry to med school was approximately 10 applicants per place. According to recent published information, in 2011, this has risen to 7-23 applicants per place. Despite rising tuition fees and increase in post-graduate debt, the medical profession is still one of the most highly sought after and desirable fields to work in. [1]

Fast forward to 2008 and to *Modernising Medical Careers* what is the modern training framework in UK medicine. In ENT the number of available places for ST3 was 19 with an average of 14 applicants per post equating to approximately 266 applicants. In 2009 there were 11 posts at national selection and 6 in London (separate selection), with a similar number of applicants, but fewer numbers available due to an obligation to honour all those awarded run through training at the time of the first MTAS scheme. In 2010, with London now included, there were 45 places with over 200 applicants, the best competition ratio yet. In 2011 there were 32 places in England, 3 in Wales, 3 in Scotland, and 1 in Northern Ireland, with more than 300 applicants. Between 2010 and 2011 training numbers were cut by 17% with most deaneries losing a training post. Currently there is a bottleneck at the post CCT stage of training for those applying for consultant posts. It has been predicted however, that by the time the current batch of new trainees come to apply for consultant posts, the pendulum will swing in the opposite direction, and there will be a reverse trend.

To become a Higher Surgical trainee in ENT then you have to start thinking and acting like one. If you can **"Walk the walk"**, then eventually you will be able to **"talk the talk"**. The way to do this is by emulating the role models in your department. Take a good look at some of the individuals in your own team; try and pick up positive traits in each member of the consultant body, write them down, and then attempt to emulate them.

These could include examples like

- He/She is a good leader
- He/She is inspirational
- He/She is very thorough
- He/She is always punctual
- This surgeon is efficient (and quick!)
- He/She is highly dedicated (to research/teaching/audit)
- He/She is a nice person (probably should be top of the list!)
- He/She is always approachable
- It is impossible to phase him/her
- He always has time for his patients and trainees

You should get in to good habits early. Come to work early, show that you are enthusiastic and keen. Try and be at least 5 minutes early, and use that to make sure everything is in place before a ward round or theatre list begins, that means knowing your patients. Be polite and kind, involve the nursing staff with your decisions and make them feel part of the team. If you are constantly late you will be at a disadvantage, your struggle will be obvious, and people will not take you seriously. Read books and journals and understand that knowledge in the right hands is a powerful tool. Write papers, reviews, audit, and contribute to book chapters. See if you can have a glance at a Consultant or Specialist Registrar's CV, it will give you an insight in to what you have to achieve in order to progress.

Dress appropriately, in other words dress as though you were a registrar in ENT. Bare below the elbows on the ward, suit, jacket or blazer for clinic, tie for meetings. Look sharp at all times, try to be clean shaven. Don't turn up to work looking a mess, in smelly dirty clothes expecting sympathy. Your colleagues and supervisors are quick to pick up on matters of tardiness and appearance and any blemishes on your character will not be forgotten easily.

A wise Consultant once declared that to succeed as a surgeon you need to have

1. The eyes of a hawk i.e. perceptive
2. The fingers of a lady i.e. dexterous
3. And the Heart of a Lion i.e. determined, strong willed and tough. Be prepared then to go that extra mile

In modern terms the characteristics of a successful surgeon could be simplified to the 3 A's.

1. **A**vailable – prepared to drop everything and help out
2. **A**ble – highly skilled and capable of performing
3. **A**ffable – likeable, personable, and able to get along with others, a good leader and team player

If you fit the mould then this means you are a kind, willing individual who is knowledgeable about their specialty, as well as being handy with surgical instruments.

If you get short listed you have to imagine that you are in a situation with people who have all the same aspirations and similar CV's to yourself. So you have to ask yourself, what makes you different and more importantly, better than those around you? This is not medical school, not everyone will make it past the post. This is the open job market and so it's you against the world.

Top tips

- Go on a few interview courses – There is a price to pay for success, but good news, it's affordable
- Know yourself – write down your strengths and weaknesses, get your friends to do the same. Evaluate, reflect, and improve

- Get consultants, and colleagues to interview you, and if you can, film the process so you and others can watch it again, be critical of your performance and improve it.
- Practice, Practice, Practice (Figure 7.6)
- Act the way you would in an interview in real life – don't just try and fake it for the day – this goes back to if you walking the walk then talking the talk.
- If you don't know the answer to a question, don't make it up, it looks bad, and if it looks like your being dishonest, it could be an instant fail! Admit your shortcomings and move on.
- Be humble. Avoid being arrogant as this will get you nowhere. The process of preparing for and attending the interview is long and frustrating, if you become short and snappy with people, you will not impress the interviewers and you will fail. Try and behave as you do on the wards and in clinic all the time, it's the recipe for success.
- Be yourself, stay calm, take your time, and eliminate words like "try" and "hope" replace with "I will do" and " I promise to…" they sound much more positive and strong. Weak language sounds horrible and interviewers will hear the positive words and will awake to find a bright enthusiastic candidate who they are ready to score highly.

Figure 7.6 Interview practice is vital before your ST3 interview

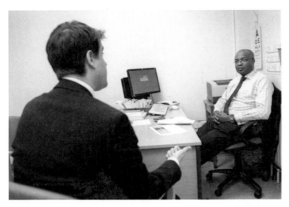

7.9 Marking scheme

In 2012, the total number of marks allocated to this station was 20. Two separate questions were asked: one question on National Guidelines and Audit, and the other on out of programme training. The marks were not equally distributed. Marks were given for an understanding of NICE guidelines on OME and the principals of audit and clinical governance, awareness of centrally appointed fellowships and the meaning of OOPE and OOPT. As much as 20 percent of the marks were allocated to global assessment of your answers, i.e., fluency, structure and organisation of answers (without too much hesitation or prompting).

Further reading

1. *Modernising Medical Careers.* Accessed via the world wide web on 24/01/2012 at www.mmc.org.uk

2.   Boyd & Fales . Reflective Learning: Key to Learning from Experience. Journal of Humanistic Psychology, *1983*

3.   Branch & Paranjape, 2002, p. 1185

4.   The Kolbs Learning cycle accessed via the world wide web on 24/01/2012 at www.brainboxx.co.uk

5.   Medical Guidelines. Accessed via the world wide web on 24/01/2012 at http://en.wikipedia.org/wiki/Medical_guideline

6.   Medical Standards of care. Accessed via the world wide web http://www.medterms.com/script/main/art.asp?articlekey=33263

7.   Medical Protocols. Accessed via the world wide we on 24/01/2012 at http://en.wikipedia.org/wiki/Medical_protocol

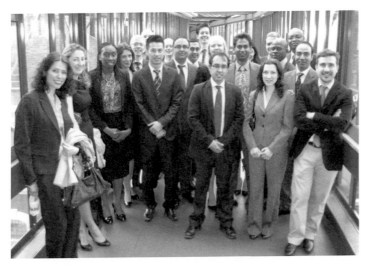

ENTTZAR Faculty members on the ST3 Interview Course 2011.